Here to Heal

Here to Heal

Reshad Feild

Element Books

© Reshad T Feild 1985
First published in Great Britain 1985 by
Element Books Ltd
Longmead, Shaftesbury, Dorset

Second impression 1986

All Rights Reserved
ISBN 0 906540 80 1

Printed by Billings, Hylton Road,
Worcester

Cover photograph by Robert Spafford
Designed by Humphrey Stone

For Penny

Contents

Introduction

In no way do I suggest that I am a healer although it is true to say that I have been able to be an instrument for healing. Over the past thirty years I have been privileged to study many methods of healing. Each of these methods has been distilled and refined within me to produce the possibility of real change in other people, change that is absolutely necessary so that they can come to see something of the purpose of life on earth.

Therapy is not necessarily real healing, although it can be a stepping-stone to awareness. True healing means the healing of the illusion that we are separate from the One Reality – a realisation that has slipped from our grasp. Healing means 'to become whole', to be one with our Creator as we were at the beginning. It is what is meant by the words in the Bible, 'to be healed of our sins', for a sin is really only a *lack,* a lack of knowledge, a state of sleep and forgetfulness. What a pity it would be if we were to pass through this life in such a state!

In our time I would like to see a ranch, called the 'Triple R Ranch', which could stand as a living example of man's responsibility to the planet and to his fellow human beings. The three R's would stand for Recognition, Redemption, and Resurrection, the three keys that unlock the door to the heart.

Our responsibility as healers is to be able to *recognise* the cause behind the cause that appears as the effect in this world, to recognise how the energy patterns work in the human body and in the land itself, and finally to recognise the hidden God that lies within each and all of us.

Redemption is the redemption of all that has prevented us from being one with the Truth itself. It is the redemption of the holding patterns that have motivated us throughout our lives for so long, our resentment, our envy and pride and all that those three walls of separation imply. In our world it takes time for life to unfold. We have time to measure the seasons, the days and nights of our lives. That which is redeemed returns to the Source of all, but it manifests in this world with the same purpose as compost has in the garden. By not allowing that which is necessary to be redeemed, we are like the person who throws away all his organic rubbish, goes out and buys an inorganic fertiliser and then complains about the cost at the supermarket! That which is redeemed makes a Garden of Knowledge for the children to come, and the children's children. Knowledge can grow out of illusion as order can stem from chaos.

Resurrection cannot come about without the apparency of death. It is said that Christ died for our sins. Yet it is also said that he never died. What apparently died was the concept of death, this little death on the stage of life, in the theatre to which we have attended from the point of conception. Something has to go for something else to enter and to transform the human being and the waiting world. What has to go, as I have said, is the illusion, so what will remain is the ever unchanging Truth that shows itself in this world of form.

The 'Triple R Ranch' would be a place where this process could occur and where people who attended there would not be afraid to be recognised for what they are, nor so scared, as so many people are, to let that which is not necessary be redeemed. They would see the purpose of the compost. They would see that the recognition and the redemption are true acts of service on their part in this great experiment we call 'Life'. They would be helping the world, for we are all interconnected, and they would know that it is good to be healed.

The Ranch would have all types of therapists, doctors,

psychologists, scientists and mathematicians. I do not see the healer as separate from the Whole. In no way do I feel that healers are an exclusive or an elitist group. Rather, I am certain, if we could only realise it, that we are all healers in our own way. What about the housewife who cooks consciously for her family and guests to help give them the strength to serve their fellow human beings better? What about the clothes designer who enhances the beauty of the woman so that all may see and notice? Then there is the carpenter who, with his craftsmanship, can influence the world for hundreds of years. The works of Chippendale and other great masters of the past are still leading us to realise that the sole purpose of Love is pure beauty. There are the architects, the stonemasons, the composers, in fact, all those who serve to bring beauty into being on earth.

History repeats itself. If we could but realise it, the quality of what has been inherently useful and good in the past can be manifested in the present. Perhaps there is a rare and beautiful painting hidden in the attic that, before this realisation, would have just remained there in its cobweb mesh. Through the 'Triple R Ranch', some memory of the faraway past might be reawakened. We might run up to the attic, recognise that indeed it was a great painting, redeem it from its present situation, get it restored if necessary and so resurrect it, bringing it to life once again.

Perhaps this Ranch is everywhere . . .

I
The Balance of Things

Solvae et coagulae, to dissolve and reform, is a great alchemical statement that bears a direct relationship to real healing. Just as each cell in the human body restructures itself every twenty-four hours, so, in a similar way, we are all potentially capable of consciously forming and reforming the patterns of our lives every day. Often we do not allow this transformation to take place and thus we carry the patterns of the past into the new day. In this way the past repeats itself, both in the outer world and in our inner being.

Most of us live in a world of habitual thinking, afraid to surrender our existing pattern lest we lose what little reality we have to cling to. Yet the future of the world lies in our hands. At this time in history, when everything is accelerating so rapidly, we are reminded to do our best to break out of these obsolete patterns that restrain us, so that we can be more adaptable to change.

Although we are partly the product of our own experiences and of the experiences of those around us, if we do dare to take a step towards real healing, beyond relative thinking and intellectual reasoning, we can grow in a new light. An entirely new set of experiences can then create in us what might be another body altogether, able, by choice, to deal with what is necessary in the many different worlds that exist within the known world. This idea, sometimes called the Body of Resurrection, has existed in the Inner Schools throughout history. Once held secret from the masses, it need not be secret any more. It is available to anyone who is willing to help to build a new world by applying all that has been useful in the past and dissolving or burning away the dross of that which is no longer needed.

Who cannot remember lying on the ground and looking up through the blue of the sky to an imaginary world of beautiful dreams? As children we have all experienced this starry world, and those of us who have been lucky enough to have been brought up in the country will remember what it felt like to live in harmony with nature itself. We trod the delicate path of natural law and if we were one of the fortunate ones, our tears were just for the washing of the eyes and not the bitter tears of grief.

Sound fixes pattern. The sound of the first seven years of a child's life forms the matrix or blueprint from which the experiences of the rest of his or her life are then built. Shocks occurring during this time can leave a lasting impression upon us. The shocks that I am referring to are not physical alone. They can also be sexual, emotional, mental motivational and aspirational. However, through order, balance, harmony and rhythm, both on the land and in the home, it is possible for a child to know the meaning of being loved.

I was born in a small village in southern England called Hascombe. It was one of those paradise places we dream about where everything is in balance and order. The village nestled in a little valley, with a forest of beech trees at the top of the hill. Stretching down to the road were acres of scarlet and white rhododendrons which people from miles around would come to see every spring. On the other side of the valley there were pastures with neat hedgerows defining the space and paths leading through the woods. As children we would take picnics and look down on the house where I was born. Originally it was a small manor house, built around 1705 in the time of Queen Anne. Later it was extended and by the time I was born, in one of the upper rooms, it was a rather large house with a superb garden spreading over several acres.

The village itself was an example of healing for everything

was as it should be. Water flowed where it was intended to flow. The different houses, having different functions, were all interconnected through the invisible worlds of which we are all a part. There were the two pubs, the village green with its maypole and the pond with the spring, where pure water gushed forth continuously, waiting for those who would come to collect it in their pails and pitchers. Harmony prevailed.

Everyone in the village knew what his or her function was both in the family and as a part of the community. I never heard of any cases of crime. No one ever locked their doors. The church was honest and there was no pretension from the vicar, though sometimes his sermons on Sundays would nearly rattle the stained glass windows when he was reminding us that we had gone to sleep yet again!

Our village midwife was also a part of the community and much respected. She lived alone and was always on call. When not delivering babies, she could be seen with her goats near the village green. She used to peg them out and then would disappear into the fields and woods, gathering herbs to make into teas for various ailments. The local doctor had a healthy respect for her too, and at Christmas people would go to her house bearing gifts. She was hardly ever known to have left the village. She was always there, ready to be of service, whether it was delivering babies or caring for the old people who needed help. The pattern of her life was a pattern of kindness, order and dignity and it had a direct effect on the whole village. I suppose she could be said to have been a natural healer.

Every time I go back to England, I visit that little village to remind me that indeed there is real hope, in living harmony, in a world where we so often see nothing but greed and chaos. As Kazantzakis said, 'It is we who are the saviours of the imprisoned God'. It is also true to say that we are all potential healers. We can be healers of the planet itself where there has been hurt and chaos. We can restore order to make a better world for our children and our children's children.

In many respects I was fortunate during my childhood. Not only were the surroundings as perfect as could be, but also it was as though some sort of guidance from a higher level brought me together with the people who then had so much influence on my life. Although sometimes we attribute this to coincidence, perhaps if we could only understand that we are given what we need for completion in this lifetime, then the people, events and settings that appear in our lives may be looked at in a new light.

Our head gardener, who stayed with the family for over thirty years, took meticulous care of the land and was a living example to everyone. I would watch him for hours as he silently went about his work, digging here, pruning there, picking up the smallest leaf that might offend the order he had created. Each morning he would come to the kitchen door with a basket laden with the fruits and vegetables he had just picked to be eaten the same day. I do not know where he was trained before he came to us, but his knowledge concerning the correct position of certain plants to protect the vegetables from bugs and beetles was extraordinary.

The shape and proportion of the various areas in the garden were worked out by the gardener and my parents. When visitors came for the weekend, they would always be invited to go for a walk through the garden before sunset, there to smell the endless combinations of perfumes from the rose garden, the hedgerows and different flower borders. It is truly amazing how our memory can retain the scent of a beautiful rose or a path lined with lavender.

The gamekeeper also had a profound influence on me. During the time we spent together on his daily rounds, he taught me the lore (law) of the land and the respect that was necessary in order to be a custodian of it. He showed me many things, one of which was how to catch a rabbit with my bare hands. By the time I was eight years old I knew nearly every step of our five hundred acres. To this day, if things were the same as then, I could walk back and point out every rabbit hole that was there nearly fifty years ago. Once during what seemed like a traumatic experience, when the gamekeeper asked me to kill the rabbit I had just caught, something happened within me which opened up a clear window into another view of the world. It was a world of free-flowing patterns, a formative world, the matrix or blueprint of this world. Perhaps it was the degree of passion and honesty in the moment that opened that window for me.

The gamekeeper's wife, tending the chickens and the geese, helped me too. She never talked to me much but would let me go around with her whilst she talked to all the chickens by the names she had given them. Each bird was taken as an individual and treated as such. The geese were trained as watchdogs for the whole estate and no one dared go near them except her. If a stranger was seen walking in the fields near their cottage, the geese would hiss and scream until she shooed them away. As a small boy I was impressed by her ability to communicate with members of the animal kingdom. It was almost as if she could speak their own language, which both understood and recognised. That was her world and from her example I would go out into the woods and try to talk to the birds there. I came to know where they roosted at night and some of them allowed me to get quite close. Again, it was a question of understanding the folk lore and natural order.

The cook was with my family for forty-seven years and woe betide anyone, including my mother, who got in her way! She taught me more, by her example of loving kindness and cleanliness, than anyone else I have ever known. To this day I pass on the knowledge I gained from her to others, who have been less fortunate than myself, in knowing the difference it makes to keep a spotlessly clean house. I can never forget the smell of her freshly starched apron, nor the time when once she came into the room when my mother was about to wop me one with the back of an ivory hairbrush. "Madam, get out!" she said. My mother fled.

When she finally died, well into her eighties, I went to pay my last respects in the little cottage we had provided for her. Her body lay so still and serene on the bed. There was no trace of any resentment, envy or pride, those three walls that divide us from the Truth. She had worked in service all her life and she was always grateful to be alive. If she had ever had any bad thoughts, they were never seen or felt. They must have been transformed into courage and overwhelming compassion for that is all we ever experienced in knowing her. I remember her presence still being in the room. It seemed to permeate me and fill my heart with gratefulness.

We all search to find some meaning and purpose in our lives. So often, though our behaviour patterns seem inexplicable, we struggle to know what has motivated us to behave in this way or that way. It takes a long time until we are able to understand that all experiences, whether viewed as positive or negative, are the greatest gifts that we are given so that we may form a true reality within ourselves. In truth, life is the only teacher. Life is made up of experiences that we are then foolish enough to judge as so called 'good' experiences or the opposite. Yet, every time we judge, it is impossible to gain a clear picture of just what any experience is trying to teach us.

Before I was sent to boarding school at the age of eight, my life was spent almost entirely out of doors. I did not like children's parties, ice cream, paper hats, sea and sandy beaches, and being virtually an only child, my half-sister already grown and gone, I had all the time in the world to explore. Although I was frequently scolded for being a loner and not liking what other children liked, I was allowed to be alone. I would go fishing by myself in the lake, or go out with the gamekeeper on his daily rounds. Just as I learned about the chickens and the geese, so I learned the different bird calls and the smell of the changing seasons. I even knew where to find the nightingale, that rare bird about whom so many poets have written, whose song sounds like living water.

However, those days were not to last. As for so many of us, certains traumas had already set up seemingly irrevocable patterns which were to motivate my actions in the future. Sometimes it takes more than one shock to activate others that have lain dormant in the subconscious.

I was not told of the first major trauma in my life until I was an adult, already married with my first son. I had always known intuitively that something had not been explained to me by my mother, she being the only person alive from my early childhood. My father had died when I was just a baby. In those days many people considered that cancer could be infectious, and it was not known that my father was already dying of cancer before I was conceived. My mother was five and a half months pregnant when this news was revealed. Everyone tightened in this moment, wondering what to do in the circumstances.

Surviving an unsuccessful abortion attempt, I finally emerged into this world weighing nearly eleven pounds. Unfortunately, I was covered with eczema over the entire surface of my body. The local doctor, a well-meaning man, advocated that I be washed daily with olive oil, that no water touch my body, and that I be placed in a muslin bag so that my small hands would not be able to touch my skin. As I said, I was not told about this incident until late in life, and my mind blocked out any memory of the fact that for the first eighteen months of my life, I was entirely enclosed in a bag! I wonder what sub-conscious motivator was created out of that experience. Perhaps I had an inbred, ever-repeating tape which activated every move of mine in the future that went something like, 'I want out of this!'

After my father died, my mother remarried twice. The first marriage did not last very long. It was during the Second World War. My stepfather was a colonel in the Home Guard which consisted of retired or semi-disabled people who could not get to the War. Since there were no rifles to speak of, he and his local brigade would march up and down on the lawn armed only with broomsticks in the hope of proper arms in the future. I would sometimes help them build tree houses along the little Surrey lanes and byways. These tree houses were intended to be a last stronghold against the expected German invasion. I believe that the men were meant to lean out from the tree houses and drop hand grenades on the advancing tanks.

It was a strange time, particularly for a young boy whose life had been so much in harmony with nature and the land. I would go and sit on top of one of the hills and watch the sky criss-cross with smoke trails as the Battle of Britain raged overhead. One after another we would see the German rockets come across from France on their way to London. Living only thirty miles from the city, we could hear the engines cut out and knew that in twenty-five seconds there would be that dreaded 'thunk' as the 'doodlebug' landed and exploded on impact. Once I went out early in the morning and found a German pilot hanging in a tree. He had been strangled by his own parachute. I remember standing and looking at him for quite a while, feeling sorry for him and wondering what his family might think.

In so many ways we are the product of our experiences. Although this period left many impressions on me, somehow or other the shocks had not seemed negative. There was a creative tension in it all. I was too young then to realise the implications of war. It had become a part of our daily lives, carried by the same voice on every wireless broadcast, announcing who had won this or that battle or how many pilots had not returned.

My mother's first divorce, in the light of the times, just

seemed like one event flowing into another. We rented a house on the South Coast where we moved until things settled down. A land mine blew up nearby during the first week we were there, shaking us all out of bed, but otherwise the time was uneventful. Eventually we moved back to our own house in Hascombe and started to put our lives in order again.

A few years later came the beginning of a crucial time in my life. I was fifteen years old, late in puberty and feeling very alone at boarding school. My mother had re-met a retired naval admiral and she came to see me at school, seeking my consent for their marriage. By the time the school term was over and I had returned to Hascombe, my mother had made the decision to sell that beloved house where I was born. The admiral wanted to live near the sea, presumably to gaze out across the ocean of his own memories. I remember the appalling pain I felt when I heard the news. Something inside me was ripped apart. What happened eventually brought me to understand why we are here on planet Earth, although it took many years of bitter resentment and pain until I could learn to be able to forgive.

I spent those twelve weeks of my summer holiday re-noting every tree on the land, consciously saying goodbye to the past. I knew somewhere inside that this event was to send me on a very long journey, perhaps away from the pain of that moment. I did not know when or even how. All I knew was that I wanted to leave that house having said farewell to every single plant, tree, bird and living creature that I had experienced in those first, formative years. When I finally got into the car with my school trunk, all dressed up in my school clothes, I asked my mother to stop at the end of the long driveway. As the car came to a halt, I stepped out and looked back one more time to say goodbye to that first portion of my life.

2

The Search Begins

We all know the sensation of 'tightening' in the moment. This may be caused by a sudden shock or fear, or by some event that we are not used to. Time gets caught in that moment and often we feel as though we have been stabbed in the solar plexus. From such experiences we can build up resentment, anger, bitterness and even grief. Instead of our memory pattern being one of loving kindness and gratitude, it is coloured by our judgements. We are caught in our opinion of what we thought should have occurred in the moment. If only we could stand back far enough to see and understand what there is to be learned from each experience, then we could turn what might appear to be negative into something positive. How many times are we veiled from such moments!

After returning to boarding school, it did not take me long to realise that, through my bitter resentment at having to leave our house, something had closed down in my heart. It was as though a blind had been pulled down over an open window. The ability I had had to see into the invisible world was taken away from me, and I felt stifled and angry, filled with dread for the future. Paradoxically, if I had not tightened during that time, I probably would not have gone on the search to find, once again, what I felt to be rightfully my own. Once we have had an inner experience of God's beauty with all of our being, it can never be forgotten.

The passion of the inner question sets our course through life. We can always be assured of one thing and that is change. If we continue to persevere in our inner yearning for the necessary changes to come about, then we can be certain that a set of circumstances will present themselves to us to provide an answer to what we need to understand in any given moment.

Shortly before my sixteenth birthday a man came to the school to give a lecture and instruction on hypnosis, or auto-suggestion. Like most boys of that age, I found such matters fascinating and signed up to go to the lecture and also to attend his classes. He only accepted those pupils who were considering a future career in the medical profession or affiliated practices. Since, at that time, I was working towards taking the necessary examinations to get me into medical school, I was invited to take the classes.

I found myself a willing and eager pupil. Even during the lecture, when certain principles were being explained to us about the practices in a rather intellectual manner, I remember that something drew me on. I felt a strange but beautiful resonance in the area of my heart when the man was speaking. Much later I discovered that he had been initiated into a high level of healing and that his methods were merely frames around the real pictures he wished us to see.

In many ways it is not the precise method in healing or therapy that really counts at all. If someone is truly able to help others up the ladder to reach a higher state of consciousness, he or she can employ a multitude of different methods, each given to suit the mentality of the patients themselves. After all, it is stated in the New Testament that even Jesus, in his Ministry, never used the same method twice!

The method that this man used was simplicity itself. He would ask us to look at a shiny object he held in his hand. He would then count to ten. By the time he had reached six or seven, we would be in the state needed to be able to work with him. Some of the pupils found this very hard in their resistance to just 'let go' into the moment, but I was fortunate. I remember that it only took two short sessions before I was able to let go of my resentment and bitterness and the window of my heart was opened once again.

Before long I was able to do the same thing. I discovered that I was perfectly capable of taking someone out of the state in which they were, whether this was physical or emotional pain, and putting them into another state, beyond the time-space relationship we have in this world. In this new state they were able to view what was going on in any one moment as though they were standing on the peak of a mountain, looking down across the valley and fields, watching what all the different people were doing.

I also discovered that those I worked with, even at that early age, were able to observe what was occurring in their own lives and to see the changing events as projections of their inner selves. It became an interesting game of pure theatre in which the participant became the director of the stage and was able to move the players into their correct roles.

Being very young, I did not realise the full significance of the part that I also was playing. I sense that it was innocence alone that protected all of us, since we had really no idea why we were playing with these methods, except that it was fun. Many other boys came to us for counselling and the fad caught on, until parents began complaining to the headmaster. One day, in a state of fear and trepidation, I was summoned to his study. He was actually a very kind and wise man and after sitting me down in a chair, soon put me at ease.

"It's all right for you to do these things if you know what you're doing, and why you are doing it. Now I am in trouble with some of the parents." He smiled then and lit his pipe. "In many ways I wish I had never invited that man in the first place. I knew him to be a good and worthwhile person and thought it could open up some things for you all. However, in the circumstances, I feel it is best that we now keep these matters to ourselves and let the flurry of excitement that has occurred since all this started die down. I will be seeing all the other boys involved individually." He continued, "I know I can trust you," and then he left the room.

The fact that I respected the headmaster so deeply enabled me to fulfil his wishes. After this talk, when people came to me to experience these phenomena, including by this time several considerably older people, I was able to say to them that I felt it was only a game and that it would be better if we played it no longer.

It would be impossible to say that what next occurred in my life was a direct result of that period, but undoubtedly something moved in me during that time. There was an opening in one of the subtle centres within me which allowed a greater flow of life force to clear the channels that had been blocked for so long. This clearing, in turn, produced even more flow.

As a child I had been granted the gift of 'second sight' into the invisible world, a gift for which I have been eternally grateful. What I 'saw' was a wondrous world of patterns in the world of nature, from which our world is continuously 'becoming'. This matrix, or blueprint, of the formative world, was like the negative of a photograph. Sometimes I would see damage in this etheric web which would then be reflected in the abnormal growth of a tree, plant, or even a human being. It was quite upsetting to me because I could see that unless something changed radically, situations could arise from that formative world which could cause hurt or damage in this world, affecting us all. At that time I never understood why other people could not see what I saw.

After my experiences with hypnosis and in using the practices to take people from one state to another, I was filled with a new type of energy which was subtly different from what I had previously known. It was as though I had another series of veins, invisible veins, patterns of endlessly moving, ever changing channels of energy, throughout my body. Sometimes I felt that I could even see them in other people. The result of this was that more than anything else I wanted to go away and truly discover what it all meant.

However, this was impossible. I was still at school and needed to remain there until the cycle was completed at the age of eighteen and a half.

Experiences are offered to us to help develop what is often called 'The Observer'. Although a portion of us is made up of the product of our experiences, we are not our experiences alone. Rather, the experiences themselves provide a mirror into which we can look, observe, and finally face ourselves. Very deep questions were arising within me during those last two years in school that I had to consider in relationship to my future. I discovered that I was not bright enough to join medical school, a bitter disappointment to my family and myself, and was therefore destined for two years compulsory service in the navy. I did not cherish the thought one little bit, but since there was no way out of it, I decided to spend any available free time studying and reading about this world of healing. As usually happens, certain books came into my hands just as they were needed and I met many gifted people who helped me along the way.

Eton College was one of the leading schools in England from which boys were prepared either for careers as officers in the army, navy or airforce, as lawyers or doctors, or in the skills needed to begin taking over their parents' estate. My newly discovered interest in healing was, in these surroundings, considered not very 'normal' either by my family or by my schoolmasters. On one occasion the family trustee was sent to see me to act as mediator, as it were, and make sure that I planned to go into business after the navy. "This hocus-pocus is all very well," he said, "but it can get you into all sorts of trouble. It is much better not to worry about such things and to concentrate instead on what your family has planned for you these past years." Oh, how much damage is done to children through their parents' expectations of them!

Genes carry the patterns of the thought-forms of our parents and ancestors. In many cases, people have little or no life of their own but live, instead, trying to fulfil the expectations that their parents have for them. The saying "Expectation is the red death", is a warning that if we expect of the child what we have not fulfilled in our own lives, the potential freedom of the essence of the child can be totally stifled. In this way, the parents are apt to be disappointed and feel a similar sense of rejection to that of the child, who only wishes to grow in the light of Truth and Freedom. Sooner or later the child will begin to overcompensate, burdened with his parents' expectations. The end result is a greater possibility that the same chaos will then be reproduced in future children, as yet unredeemed from the patterns of the past.

My inner questions during this period were far deeper than my considerations about the family business. They were concerned with the nature of time and the deep inner meaning of religion, not in its formal sense *per se,* but rather the functions of the different religions at various periods of history and in different parts of the world. The formative worlds that I had been experiencing were not subject to the laws of our world of time and space, and yet they were just as real to me as watching the seasons change at their due time in this world. I read about the idea of eternal recurrence and spent hour upon hour just sitting in the sixteenth century school chapel, sensing what still remained in the present time from the worshippers who had gone long ago.

At times, the presence of Christ was so overwhelming in the chapel that I went to the school chaplain to ask his advice. I explained that often I felt tears welling up inside me and how, after each occasion there would be a sense of release which defied all normal understanding. The chaplain was a kind and gentle man. Convinced that my future was to lie in the formality of a church structure he advised that I go to a theological college. This was to be my work in life, he said, in gratefulness for all that I'd been given to experience. By the time that I finally left school, we had spent many hours together in prayer and contemplation. Although it was a sad parting, by then the chaplain had guessed, and rightly so, that my life was to be in the streets and not in the Church alone.

3
Synchronicity and the Path of Return

As our understanding of healing grows, a series of events almost inevitably occurs in our lives which cannot be explained by chance alone. The laws governing synchronicity are difficult, if not impossible, to understand with the logical mind. The mind thinks along a pathway that goes from point A through point B to point C, whereas synchronicity has very much to do with the Path of Return, the path we have taken to return through life's experiences to the Source of Life itself.

There are hundreds of stories that can be told in which events seem to take place for no logical reason. We have all had such experiences at different times of our lives. I have found, over the years, that these strange events occur to guide us along the way, when we are really living in a question. If we just presume life and let things take their normal course, we may not notice what is really going on around us. We see and experience only what we want to, rather than what we might need. On the other hand, if there is a question burning in our hearts, then life takes on a totally different meaning. A stranger passing by us on a street corner may carry the whole answer to the mystery in a glance. If we are asleep to the moment, the event will mean absolutely nothing and we will lose another opportunity which could help us piece together the jigsaw puzzle of our life's journey.

In a sense, all life in the relative world has to do with healing. With this understanding, there is a new and different meaning to that which we so often view as suffering in ourselves and in others. Each moment can be a healing experience for we are never given more pain that we can bear. All that we are given has inevitably to do with the possibility of self-transformation. Everything, whether perceived consciously or not, is part of this transformation process. If we are asleep to the great potential that we, as human beings, have within us, then we are only a part of organic evolution. If we are awake to our purpose in life's journey, then we are participating in the conscious evolution of mankind and of the future of the planet itself.

The time that I spent in the navy was, to say the least, eventful, and the laws of synchronicity worked very strangely indeed. I was commissioned as a navigating officer, but this later proved to be an unsuccessful choice on the part of those in command. I still have the reputation of being the only person who managed to navigate a squadron of motor-torpedo boats into a minefield in peacetime!

My career at sea was thus short-lived and I was transferred instead into naval intelligence. Had this not been the sequence of events I might never have learned to type, then a compulsory skill for those of us decoding foreign signals, and one which today is still invaluable to my work. I was also granted plenty of spare time on the job, which I took advantage of to renew my studies in esoteric healing. The further I delved into the mysteries, the more I realised that there was no end to what could be learned.

The search was on again and I used every spare moment for study. The Prophet Mohammed once coined the famous saying, 'Seek ye Knowledge even unto China', and in those days China was a long way from Medina! And so I continued. Every now and again I would have glimpses of that 'Real World' I used to know as a child and which had been concealed from me ever since. People began coming into my life, even at that young age, who wanted my help, and I found that they were able to receive it. My hands would get red hot as I touched the afflicted parts of their bodies and sometimes a breath of cool air would enter the room where I was working. I also used what I had assimilated in school about auto-suggestion and adapted it intuitively to the moment.

After these experiences, I could hardly wait to be released from the navy. The last six months dragged on and on. By that time my family had made plans for me to join the stock exchange and to work in the city of London, all of which seemed utterly distasteful. The stock market did not add up to my concepts of what healing was all about. I was much more concerned with being of real service in my life. Although I did end up going to a stockbroker's office after taking off my officer's uniform, I only lasted three weeks. 'I want out of all this' was the ever-running theme through my heart and mind.

Something was drawing me on and out of the traditional background I had been so used to. In those days youth was not on the move very much and I was essentially on my own. This was in the fifties, long before the great youth revolutions of the sixties and seventies. In England, the few of us who were the discontented youth were termed 'angry young men'. We caused a great deal of havoc wherever we went and spent much of our time in intellectual left-wing activities.

In all the rebellious glamour of the avant-garde during that period, I nearly forgot my main purpose, which was to recommit myself continually to the search for Truth. Then, once more, I realised that there was nothing else I could do. Destiny drew me on. For no logical reason that even I, at that time, knew, and much to my family's displeasure, I took out emigration papers for the United States of America.

Approaching New York and seeing the Statue of Liberty for the first time in the early morning light, it really did seem that I was one of the pioneers from the days of *The Mayflower,* I could hardly wait to reach the shore. My enthusiasm didn't last very long, however, as the impressions of the city soon became overwhelming. Everything was so noisy, so busy and so frenetic and I felt far away from the quietude of the English countryside. After a few days I found the commotion unbearable and decided to move on.

I went by train to North Carolina. The impressions I had of the deep South triggered off all the stories I had heard about the American side of my family. Bishop Feild was one of the first bishops to come to America. He was a descendant of Sir John Feild, the court astronomer to Queen Elizabeth I, who granted him a knighthood in 1538. Sir John Feild was known to be a great expert on Copernicus's mathematics and was an acquaintance of John Dee, the famous occultist who founded The Golden Dawn, an inner esoteric society which exists to this day. Together, Sir John Feild and John Dee worked out the route for Sir Francis Drake to sail around the world.

North Carolina was where my ancestors had lived for generations. I wanted to get a sense of my roots since there was no knowledge of anyone else in the Feild family being so totally immersed in the inner quest after the sixteenth century. Do we not all have a desire to trace our ancestry? We carry so much of the pattern of the past. To be free, as healers of the world, it is important that through Love, we distil the patterns of the unfulfilled love of the generations that have gone before us.

I was shocked to find the family estate run down. The once beautiful colonial house had been neglected for years, and my only living relative was an aged cousin whose main desire was that I immediately marry one of the local débutantes. I was given parties galore and young women were lined before me as though I was going to pick one of them like a spring flower!

It was all too embarrassing but since humour has a great part to play in healing, I will relate the following Zen-like story. I was pursued day and night by eager mothers wanting a Feild back in North Carolina, and found little opportunity to escape. As a last resort, I announced that I was very keen on fishing and made myself a fishing rod. Then, armed with a cork, a long piece of string, a bent pin and a small worm, I repaired to the local pond. Even there I was not allowed to be alone and people began arriving to stare at this apparition. I had already been informed that there were no fish in the pond. Finally, one of the locals asked me why I baited my hook when everyone, including myself, knew that there were no fish to be caught. I replied, "But if I do not bait the hook, how will I know that there are no fish?" My ploy was successful in, as it were, getting me off the hook! Not only did they understand that I had no intention of marrying one of the glamorous southern belles but they had also decided, by that time, that I was a bit crazy. I was left alone, at last, to contemplate my roots and to decide what my next step would be.

Eventually I landed up in Memphis, Tennessee, where I worked in the office of a cotton magnate for several months, in exchange for a plane ticket to Japan. My journeys in America seemed to have served their purpose and I felt that it was soon time for me to leave. Whether he liked my British accent or whether my secretarial abilities were better than I thought, I was given, much to my surprise, not just a plane ticket to Japan, but one around the world. Although I never saw the man again, by some strange quirk of fate or destiny and through the laws of synchronicity, I was able to continue my journey.

From Memphis, I boarded a plane to San Francisco. There I was a stranger in a strange land once again, wearing my tweed suit, which was really made for the Scottish moors, and carrying only my guitar and an enormous suitcase. In those days, San Francisco represented a pathway to freedom, particularly for those people who had found themselves enmeshed in a stoical English society. The cable cars, the music, the laughter and the over-all sense of joy, were almost too tempting for me to leave.

We all need three types of food every day: the food we

eat, the air we breathe, and the impressions we take in. Without all three, there can be little *real* life. Impressions are necessary and need to be consciously gathered, rather than just presumed. No two moments are the same and so the pathway we tread one day is never the same as the one before, or the one to come. After having spent all my time in an office in Memphis, I feasted on the impressions in San Francisco, and by so doing, felt a sense of healing.

My next step was to Hawaii. Oh, what incredible glamour in those days! Heaven opened up to a young Englishman. The tweed suit was discarded on the beaches of Waikiki, and mai tai cocktails took the place of the proverbial cup of tea. I felt like one of the sailors with Captain Cook when he first landed in Tahiti. Gone were my aims for Truth and my aspirations to learn about healing in order to be more of service. Gone were the high ideals. Nothing existed but an endless world of sensual attraction.

If we get caught in the world of attraction, we are apt to lose our way, and yet it is attraction itself that draws us on. As we go out on this journey to return to the Essence of Truth itself, then every experience we have been given can be seen as a signpost to guide us along the road. There is no blame if we miss the sign the first time, or the second, or third, but if we continually ignore what we are given to understand, then surely it will be difficult for us to see the purpose of the next test. Truth is not delivered on a silver salver but is distilled within from hard work and good observation.

Because the question in my heart was real, I was guided, though sometimes in 'Paddington Bear' fashion, along the Road of Truth. Even in Hawaii, surrounded by all its pleasures, certain events happened that woke me up once again to my original intention. As a result, I re-established my plans to travel to Japan. In school I had read about Zen Buddhism, studied Japanese art and had always felt drawn to the serenity of the countryside there. I also knew, intuitively, that it held a key to my search.

Unfortunately, I had not sufficiently learned from my experiences in Hawaii about how the world of attraction can appear to deflect us from our aim and so something similar happened to me on the plane to Japan. I met a very beautiful air hostess on the flight. We decided that we liked each other a lot, and before I left the plane, she gave me a piece of paper with the name of her hotel in Kyoto, where we were to meet again in three days' time. For some reason, between my completing certain matters in Tokyo and arriving in Kyoto, I lost the little piece of paper with the address of the hotel. I was eager to meet her there, as romance was afoot! Disappointed, I tried my best to look back into that time on the aeroplane and finally I thought that I remembered the name of the hotel. Woe betide the people who 'think' that they know!

The train from Tokyo to Kyoto was very crowded. I still carried my enormous suitcase and guitar, but luckily now travelled with some lighter clothes. Arriving in Kyoto, I asked for a taxi and tried to explain to the taxi driver where I wanted to go. He spoke not a word of English, and I not a word of Japanese. He looked rather strangely at my request to go to this particular 'hotel'.

Driving at breakneck speed until he turned off the main road, and then winding around the back streets, he finally stopped in a narrow lane outside a large wooden door. Trying his best to explain in sign language, he motioned that this was the address that I had given him. He seemed in a great hurry and as soon as I had paid his fare, he drove off. I was left alone, standing in the street with my guitar and my suitcase.

We all know that tingling feeling we get when something is about to happen. There is a sensation in the nape of the neck, and it balances with a little fear right in the solar plexus. Well, I had just that. By now it was fairly obvious that this could not be the hotel that had been written on that little slip of paper. Somehow 'Paddington' had done it again.

I knocked on the door. It was opened by three young women in dark silk kimonos who, smiling, led me into quite one of the most beautiful Japanese gardens I had ever seen. No photograph could do it justice. The sense of order, peace and tranquility took away all my fears. I felt as though I were at home again in Hascombe, even though I was in another country. There was the same sense of purpose. Even a garden can be a healer.

The young women, who I discovered later were novitiates indicated that I was to wait by the doorway. Despite my fear being melted in the beauty of the garden, I really did feel that I must be somewhat out of my mind. I had no idea where I was. The shock of the situation changed time. The young women were incredibly beautiful and attractive but there was no sign of hotel rooms or anything that resembled a hotel. I remembered the face of the taxi driver when he left me at the door. Was this a brothel? What strange circumstances had I found myself in this time?

I could see a portion of a long, low building that seemed to be almost part of the garden. There was no separation. Everything was in perfect proportion and harmony. I sat on top of my suitcase and waited, feeling entirely out of my depth. In a short while the young women returned, this time joined by a monk in robes. He had a shaved head, and carried what looked like a flattened stick in his hands. He bowed deeply and was able to speak just enough English for me to ascertain that I was in a monastery. In fact, it turned out to be a Zen Buddhist monastery where the novices learned about the ancient art of the Tea Ceremony.

The laws of synchronicity were at work again. I later discovered that I had pronounced one syllable in the name of the hotel incorrectly. As a result, I ended up spending the next few weeks in the monastery, quietly meditating with the others there, receiving instruction from the Abbot, and experiencing the healing properties of the order and pattern that prevailed in the house and garden.

During my stay, it became increasingly clear to me that the importance of the correct use of pattern in healing is so often overlooked. The healing properties of sacred architecture or of a correctly laid out garden can never be overstressed. No one can ever be quite the same after being in a Gothic cathedral or somewhere like the Blue Mosque in Istanbul. How much more care and consideration would we take in building our gardens, homes and cities if we knew that even the damage caused by shocks and emotional stress can be mended by just being in such places.

Throughout that period, I seemed to live in a series of flashbacks to the time I spent as a child. The pain of moving from the house where I was born began to melt away and that inner sight again became available to me. With that gift also came the growing realisation that somehow or other I would start a healing centre in England. I had no idea how this would come about, nor indeed when, but the groundwork was being laid. As I sat in that beautiful monastery garden, I had visions of a place where people could come, where therapeutic work could be given to those in need, and where harmony and order could be restored to those coming from the cities. Many years went by before that vision materialised, but I am convinced that those weeks had a profound effect on me, once again renewing my endless quest for Truth.

The time came for me to move on. The day that I planned to leave, the Abbot arranged for the full Tea Ceremony to be given. Despite the language difficulties and the fact that I could not understand the significance of all the movements, it was a powerful and moving experience. Our parting was a fond one. I can never forget the kindness and generosity of those dear, gentle people.

I never did meet up with the air hostess again, but all that I gained from the monastery made it hardly seem like a loss. It was there that I also learned the basic principles of conscious breathing. The Abbot used to tell me again and again, "You remember please. You breathe in only to breathe out." Over the next years I spent long periods in various types of meditation and learned many techniques from different teachers, but I always came back to that first principle as I do to this day. With the conscious use of breath and through balancing our 'in-breath' with our 'out-breath', a whole new world is made available to us.

4
Journeys to the East

It is extraordinary how, just when we think that everything is going our way and life seems easy and flowing beautifully, something comes in, apparently through chance, to disturb the pattern. Our plans are turned upside down and we wonder what went wrong and why we had to start all over again. When we are young, it is difficult to understand that our experiences provide us with the food for growth. If we are grateful for the experiences and all that they bring, then we can proceed and other, greater sources of food are then offered to us.

The time I spent in Japan was healing in so many ways, but I had no real aim as yet. My journey on the road towards Truth had led me through many rich experiences but I now needed a 'frame' through which I could apply all that I had been given to understand. Without this frame, I knew that I had to return to England and face the inevitable boredom of the life which I had been brought up to accept as being normal. I did not relish the thought. I wondered how I could fit into society once more and follow the rounds of cocktail parties, dinners, and balls that were so in vogue at that time. The idea of a dinner suit seemed totally incongruous and black, patent-leather shoes were a far cry from a Japanese monastery!

After leaving Tokyo, I went to Hong Kong and tried to gather myself together to face western culture once again. I played tennis at the British club there, attended numerous parties that were entirely British and, within a short space of time, ended up thoroughly bored. My old tape of 'I want out of this!' was playing loudly inside and, because I had enough money to avoid the whole issue, I flew to India, and then on to Pakistan. It was there that the inevitable shock came. I contracted such a severe case of amoebic dysentery that I had to return to England, where I found myself in a London hospital. Complications in my health occurred there and I spent much of the next few years in and out of different hospitals, undergoing a serious operation, and generally speaking, getting about as fed up as anyone could with orthodox medicine.

Like so many others, I began to see that if the medical profession were to work hand in glove with the various healers and therapists of the world, there could be a great breakthrough in the understanding of health and disease. At that time, I decided to work in a hospital myself, in order to be of service and to learn more about suffering and death. Because my family knew the then executive head of one of the largest teaching hospitals in London, I managed to get a job there. I befriended many doctors. Gone were the plans for me to become a stockbroker, a brewer or a rich business-man. I was on my own now, and set on the idea of one day opening a true centre of healing, working hand in hand with the orthodox medical profession, with a team to help in every level that was possible. I saw chiropractors, osteo-paths, herbalists and many other therapists all working together. The dream was far-fetched, but eventually it did come to pass.

I was invited, at one point, to go to Ajmer, India, to deliver a series of lectures on esoteric healing. At the last moment something inside shouted so strongly to me that I was not to go, that I cancelled the tour and changed my plane tickets to fly to Karachi in Pakistan instead. I planned to stay with my cousin there, although I had not seen him since I was a child and had no idea of the sort of life he led. The country club setting in which I found him was in strong contrast to the rampant poverty of the ghettos nearby. On some days the stench of suffering and starvation would waft on to the grounds, though it was met with little compassion from those rich enough to buy their way out of pain. If we are 'One Brotherhood of Man in the Fatherhood of God', but cannot remember the pain of our brothers and sisters, then we can hardly call ourselves human. I stayed only a week or so with my cousin, and then, led by an even stronger question as to the purpose of life on earth, I set off to the northern part of Pakistan.

I had seen many pictures of the northern territories above Rawalpindi, close to the Afghanistan border and had read about that mysterious place called Hunza, where the people live to be well over a hundred. Knowing full well that I was on the verge of a great change in my life, I looked forward to having time to sit quietly for a while, and the thought of those beautiful mountains drew me on. I had to wait in Rawalpindi because the weather was too bad for the small plane to make the incredible journey to Gilgit, nearly 5,000 feet up in the Himalayas. Eventually it cleared and we took off. Gone were the days of the huge suitcase, guitar and tweed suit. This time it was a backpack, warm clothes, and a portable stove!

At that time, the army was concerned about the Chinese coming through that area *en route* to Pakistan. As a result, visitors were only allowed to stay in the government rest houses and were asked to travel by jeep with a specially appointed government driver. I had not expected this. I had very much hoped to just be on my own and let the future unfold. The flight was one of the most hair-raising of my life, with the wings nearly scraping the sides of the huge, soaring mountain peaks way above us. When the plane did safely land, I was whisked away to the only rest house in the area, and issued with the necessary special visitor's papers.

I rested in the guest house for a few days, cooking the food that I had brought on the little stove outside my room on the verandah. The restaurants looked suspicious and I wasn't willing to take any chances, remembering my bouts

of dysentery in Pakistan those years ago. As there was no
one else staying at the house it was quiet, and a good time
for me to take stock.

When I finally felt acclimatised to the height and thoroughly settled, I went out to explore the town and market
place. It was there that I noticed a man selling cloth. An
instant recognition took place on both sides and he invited
me into the tiny shop for tea. He had piercing eyes, spoke
fluent English, and was incredibly polite and dignified,
despite his somewhat ragged appearance. After a few pre-
liminaries, he started asking me question after question
about my life. He wanted to know what I was doing all
alone in Gilgit, where I had been in Pakistan and so on. It
was not long before we got on to the matter of my own
personal search for Truth, and the idea that we are all here to
heal in one way or another. The conversation went on all
day. In the evening, he invited me to his house and sent a
boy running to forewarn his wife that there was a guest for
dinner.

The small house was just a short walk away. The man
took my arm and steered me through the crowds. In those
days, few foreigners visited Gilgit and so I was stared at in
no uncertain way. People even came running out of the side
streets to have a look at this phenomenon. I was glad to have
my tailor friend with me, who shooed away those who
came too close. We were greeted by his wife and eldest
daughter, who were both wearing the most exquisite silk
clothes. I was treated royally, and the meal that they prepared has remained in my memory ever since. There were
many dishes, each one subtly flavoured, but what I remember most was the rice. It was covered in pure silver foil as
thin as rice paper. "If I had had more notice, it would have
been gold," the wife said, with a smile, signifying that I was
to eat it along with the rice.

Dinner came and went, more questions were asked, and
then the women left and we talked over tea. As always

happens in the Middle East, if people from the West begin
to ask questions about the Inner Path, inevitably the subject
of Sufism comes up. Sufism is the esoteric core of Islam and
something that I had been studying in depth in London. In
any orthodox religious background, these subjects are seldom discussed openly. I had been given more than a faint
hint that this humble man knew more about it than he was
prepared to tell at that first meeting. There is nothing like a
good bait to catching a willing fish and so the next day, I
was back at his shop!

On that particular day, the tailor was busy, but he had
arranged for me to see a friend of his. Before I left, though,
he insisted on measuring me, saying that he wanted to
present me with a gift when I returned the next morning.
The friend in question turned out to be a rug seller on
another street. Again, a similar situation developed with
many cups of tea and more questions. Because he did not
speak English very well, this time the questions were more
difficult to answer. He explained to me that he had spoken
with his friend, the tailor, who told him that I was interested
in the healing arts. He went on to say that he had a friend
further north who knew about these matters and, if I were
going that way, I might be able to meet him. As there was
no address, he drew me a rough map, and explained that
still further on was a government rest house at the foot of
Nanga Parbit, the 'Naked Mountain', 8,000 feet higher than
where we were in Gilgit.

The next morning I returned to my friend the tailor at his
shop. "I am so honoured that you have come," he said, and
then, going to the back, he brought out a magnificent
woollen robe. "It will keep you warm," he said, smiling. "I
would have made a lining for it as well, but the only material
I had is the little I have put inside the cuffs. Please take it and
remember us when you are high up in the mountains. I have
heard about your plans and have arranged for a government
driver to pick you up tomorrow. You must take some food

with you, enough for at least a week, for the driver will not
stay where you are going, and you must be well prepared.
May Allah guide you safely on your journey.''

How often have we been told to trust, and yet how seldom are we ever told that trust is of such a high quality, that
it is not in just trusting one human being or in a set of
circumstances, but rather, being in a state of trust, which in
itself allows what is necessary to come forth in the relative
world. Living in a state of trust produces an understanding
of synchronicity.

I did find the healer but I felt that it was more by luck than
good judgement. The rough map that I had been given
made little sense to the jeep driver, who spoke no English at
all. After we had driven for a short while, the road turned
into a narrow dirt track, hardly wide enough for the jeep to
get through. People were working in the fields but otherwise there was nothing to be seen except for the towering
mass of mountain rising into the sky.

We must have gone about halfway when I saw a man
walking ahead of us. He had long black hair, which is very
unusual in that part of the world, and he immediately
caught my eye. He was wearing a robe similar to my own,
which I had carefully packed with my other clothes. Behind
him walked a boy of about fourteen years of age, carrying a
bundle of juniper branches in his arms. Juniper, I later
discovered, when made into a tea, is an excellent tonic,
particularly for women. If it is burnt in the fire grate first
thing in the morning, juniper also has the property of
clearing the room of left-over thought forms from the day
before.

Asking the driver to stop, I stepped out and approached
the man. For a while he seemed suspicious, and because I
spoke no language known in that area, and he not a word of
English, I was surprised when he suddenly beckoned me to
follow him down a little path. The driver refused to come
along and stayed with his jeep.

We walked in single file. Rounding a bend, we came upon a small hut. A group of about fifteen was gathered in a clearing in front, sitting on the rocks and on the ground. Immediately they all stood up to greet this strange man and the boy. At first, they would not look at me, but then, one by one, they warmed up and I was accepted. A fire was being made in the clearing. The man went into the hut and then, after the boy had put the juniper branches on top of the fire, came out again. There was chanting, and then the man knelt and bent forward, catching the smoke in his hands and inhaling it deeply. After a while, he stood up again and took a stick in his hand. One by one the people came up to him and he would make a pattern in the sand at his feet. He then placed a glass of water in the pattern for each individual, said some prayers, and then gave the water to that person to drink.

It became obvious then that all these people were suffering from some ailment or another and that he was the local healer. I heard later that people came from miles around to see him, and that when he breathed in the juniper smoke, he could see into another, formative world and thus diagnose each particular ailment. The effect of the patterns that he made in the sand went in turn into the water, which then became the remedy for the sick person.

Many healers use methods similar to that used by the man in Pakistan to diagnose the cause of an illness that has manifested in the relative world. Once, in Turkey, I saw a similar type of person using molten lead. He would melt the lead in a pan over the fire whilst holding the patient's hand and then empty it into a bowl of water. The cold of the water would immediately form the lead into a pattern. When it was cool enough, he would take it out and explain what he saw was wrong with the person from the pattern of the lead. Those early experiences led me on, further and further, to study the nature of pattern, and were invaluable in helping me to understand how to interpret the formative worlds. There are so many worlds within worlds.

I bade farewell to that strange gathering, and found the jeep driver still standing by the side of the road waiting for me. We continued, ascending the dirt track until we finally came into an area where there was a pasture. The track ended there and, just behind some pine trees, the rest house stood firmly. It seemed it had been there for years. Probably it had been a mountain hut for climbers before the political turmoil that had broiled up after the war.

As he helped me out of the jeep with my portable stove and back-pack, my driver managed to explain that he would come back in seven days' time. Hardly turning round, he got back into the jeep and sped off down the track. It was late in the afternoon and the glaciers above me were just starting to turn pink in the setting sun. For a while I stood, watching all the wonder of those mountains, and tried to get acclimatised to the rarified atmosphere. I was now at 12,500 feet and it was hard to breathe. As I settled into the present moment, after the long drive, I became aware that I was not alone. Although the sun had not yet gone down and so there were no lamps lit in the rest house, I could sense that someone was there. Knocking on the door, I heard movement within and then out came a woman and her husband, who turned out to be Scottish missionaries on a bird watching vacation . . . What more unlikely situation could occur way up there in the Himalayas! "Would you like a cup of tea?" the woman asked, as though this was all absolutely normal.

We talked together until it was time to light the lamps. Suddenly there was a knock on the door. "Now who would that be?" asked the lady in her broad Scottish accent. The door opened and in walked a tough looking man with a huge back-pack and an ice-pick. "My name is Hans," he said. "Is it all right if I stay the night?" Hans, it turned out, was a professional climber, German by birth, who had been on one of the Everest expeditions. He had just climbed across Afghanistan, which, at that time, was totally illegal,

and was preparing to ascend the huge mountain that tower-
ed above us, now made silver by the moon.

The stories went on late into the night but we were all up
early in the morning to see the sunrise. Directly after breakfast, when the Scottish couple told us of their plans for the
day, Hans asked me if I would like to go climbing with him.
For some unaccountable reason I agreed. The absurdity of
this was that I was afraid of heights, had no really suitable
clothes or climbing boots, and the fact that he intended to
take me up to a glacier at 15,000 feet where the air is thin
indeed!

We climbed and climbed, up the steep shale slopes. It was
slippery and dangerous without proper boots, and yet,
despite my fear, on I went. At one point, I completely lost
my nerve and could neither go up nor down. I called for
help. Hans, although physically strong, was not very tall,
but he managed to pull me up the slope. Eventually we
arrived at the glacier. It was one of the most beautiful sights
I had ever seen, with Nanga Parbat to our left, as we looked
down over the valley. We could just see the rest house 3,000
feet below. Resting, we shared some water together and
Hans told me some of his climbing adventures. By now, I
was suffering from altitude sickness and snow blindness and
was a bit worried about what to do. Suddenly, Hans stood
up on the ice and announced that he was climbing on to
make his first camp on the ascent, and that I was to return to
the rest house alone. I was speechless, absolutely terrified,
but there was nothing that I could do about the situation.
We shook hands and parted. Reluctantly, I watched his
small frame move on up the glacier until I could see him no
longer.

Calling on my past experience and knowledge, I closed
my eyes and breathed quietly in order to calm myself. I
could not have been sitting there long when suddenly, as
though on a television screen, a picture unfolded in front of
me. I saw an old derelict farm in England that I had never
seen before, with a small river running through the valley

just below the main house. Abruptly, the scene changed and I saw the farm converted into a healing and teaching centre. I saw people with light in their eyes, happily working in the gardens. A wonderful air of joyous peace permeated everything and I remembered what I had sensed in that beautiful garden in the Japanese monastery.

When I opened my eyes again, I was filled with a sense of wonder and glorification. With no further ado, I started down the mountain, and this time I was not at all afraid. I returned to the house to wait for the driver to come back in six days' time and to meditate on what had occurred. Although I never saw Hans again, the Scottish bird watchers stayed for two more nights.

During the week it became obvious to me what I now had to do. The farm was somewhere in England and I had a very strange sensation that I knew just where it could be found, even though I had never been to that part of England before. If my intuition was correct, somehow or other I would turn it into the healing centre I had seen on the glacier, way up there in northern Pakistan. Before I left, I vowed that I would do everything I could to find that farm. It was an undertaking about which, by this time, I had little or no choice.

5
The Farm is Found

There is a great saying from the Sufi tradition: 'Keep your intention before you at every step you take. You wish for freedom and you must never forget it.' And yet, what is the 'freedom' that we are asked to remember? Seldom are we taught all that this word implies. We can have 'freedom' from something. We can have 'freedom' in moving towards our destination, having already been freed of the compulsions that drove us on for so long. We can also have 'freedom' in the knowledge that it is this very freedom we wish for, not for ourselves alone, but for our children and our children's children.

I carried my vision of the farm home with me to London, feeling a strange sense of urgency to share it. After unpacking, I telephoned the friends with whom I had meditated on a regular basis for many years and we arranged to meet at once. As we had spent many hours in the past talking about the chances of starting a centre, they were very interested in hearing what had transpired on the glacier. Perhaps we were just on the verge of seeing our dreams come true.

It is so easy to forget our original intention and to get diverted into doing something we did not plan to do at all. Luckily my friends and I remembered the qualities needed to fulfil the undertaking we were about to begin, qualities of trust, courage, rhythm, perseverance, faith and also of respect, in the knowledge that, as John Donne wrote, 'No man is an island...'

The people in the meditation group came from all walks of life and followed varied professions. One of the men, an antique dealer, lived in the country and my inner sense was that, if the farm really did exist, it was in his direction. We took out a map of the area, noting where farms were mentioned, and resolved to spend any available time driving around, searching for anything that might resemble what I had seen. We asked in the village pubs if the local farmers knew of such a place, questioned in the post offices and inquired at the police stations. For a while there was no clue. Perhaps my vision was merely a case of snow blindness after all.

One day I received a call from my antique dealer friend. "I think I've found it," he said. "It's about ten miles from my house." He went on to describe it and virtually everything seemed to fit in with the rough drawing that I had made for them. I told him I would leave London immediately and would meet him at his house. Taking another friend with me, I set off. I believe I was shaking a little with the anticipation of it all.

It was the place! There was absolutely no doubt about it. The main house was there, the barns and even the little river which flowed through the valley. It was more beautiful than I had imagined, in spite of its derelict state. Some of the old roofs had fallen in, the inside of the house was damp and there were many leaks. The river was clogged and if there had once been a garden, there was no sign of it any more. Although everything was totally overgrown with grass and weeds and there were few birds around, all I could see was possibility. As we explored every nook and cranny, I could already envision people walking along the pathways through the gardens and could hear children laughing and playing.

The agent informed us that the farm had been empty for the past four and a half years. Originally it was the farmhouse for a much larger acreage, but several farms locally had formed a syndicate and thus there was no more use for it as a farmhouse. How on earth no one had bought it in the meantime will always remain a mystery. It was almost as though, through some strange act of destiny, it had waited for that moment when we agreed to buy it. Pooling our resources, we wondered just what we had let ourselves in for.

It was not by chance that during the following years, as the derelict buildings began to be transformed, I met up with the man who was to become my spiritual teacher.* It is said that when the pupil is ready, the master will come. I am fully convinced that it is only in dedicating ourselves to a life of conscious service for the future of humanity and indeed the planet itself that we truly meet up with the right person who can bring about the necessary transformation in our own lives.

The farm did become a healing centre. People came from all over the world to help build this place which offered such objective hope. We started work on the big house first, mending the roof and making it habitable enough for people to sleep on mattresses on the floor. There was only one bathroom for everyone. The kitchen was minute and had it not been for the willingness of all the visitors, the work would never have been possible. As it was, people pulled together, working from sunrise to sunset, in extremely difficult conditions. Before long, work had also begun on one of the barns, to provide dormitory space, since the main house was now bursting at the seams.

Healing takes place on so many levels. Although some people might have felt that until the centre was physically complete and ready to receive guests, it could not fulfil its intended function, the truth of the matter was that it was just as much the building of the centre and the residential study courses held at the same time, that enabled balance and harmony to exist. Every individual had a function. There was always physical work to be done, for all ages, as well as the study groups and periods of meditation. Everything worked together to balance the physical, mental and aspirational parts of the being.

*See *The Last Barrier*, Element Books.

The farm continued to grow into our vision. In the first year a small garden was laid out which was extended later to make one big enough to provide sufficient vegetables for the whole community. The visitors poured through the gates every weekend, some staying for periods of up to six months. In the second year we converted a stable block into single and double rooms and, at last, managed to have nine bathrooms and shower units. In the second year we also erected a huge dome inside the great sixteenth century cruciform barn. It was like a pearl within the heart of an oyster, supported on nine huge oak pillars which we all had a hand in sanding and polishing. Each pillar itself had nine sides.

During those years, people were truly happy and a great number received the healing they needed. The land too was healed. The river was cleared so that it flowed freely once more. We planted an orchard of four hundred apple and pear trees and the birds returned. Money appeared when it was needed so that, although we were never wealthy, we always managed to get by. If we are clear about our aim, and hold a question in our hearts, then we are the pupils of the moment and things do fit into place in some strange way.

In the light of synchronicity, I suppose it was not surprising for us to discover that our sixteenth century farm happened to be built on a much older building. When we first began the restoration plans, in many places we had to dig down deep into the earth. In one spot we went down about fifteen feet and still the stone wall continued downwards. There the stones were cut much thinner. Through this method, it was possible for us to date what were the original buildings to around the ninth or tenth century. Putting two and two together, we understood, and later confirmed, that the farm had been built on top of what had once been a monastery which, like so many hundreds of others, had been sacked in the sixteenth century.

For many years I had been studying the nature of sacred places on the planet and of certain special spots which had always served as places of pilgrimage, long, even, before Christianity came to England. Churches were built on these spots and it seemed, in my research, that there was a vortex of healing force held in the very land itself. In my work I had visited many such places around the world and recognised their importance. It could not have been by chance that our cruciform barn had been constructed on top of one of these vortices.

In the dome, inside the barn, we performed sacred movements on the same spot that had been used for sacred purposes for hundreds of years. To meditate there was healing, and people would travel from far and wide to come inside and sit quietly. Indeed, the land itself is a great healer if we know where to go. If the seal of the ancient wisdom is opened to us, we will know the correct place upon which to build, for our children and our children's children.

We did see our dream to completion. Even as times changed and the need for that particular aspect of the work of transformation was no longer necessary, the beauty of the land remained as a testimony to the love and care of those times. Eventually the farm was sold, and today, with little alteration, it provides a series of cottages and flats for people coming from the cities to obtain the quiet benefit of that beautiful place. Some of the people who had been involved felt that because the centre did not continue as it was, it was a failure. However, it is always important to adapt to the times in order to discover how best to be of service. The farm today is providing exactly what is necessary.

The work of transformation goes wherever it is needed and appears in different ways. Often it is disguised so that form does not creep in to turn the fluidity of the moment into blind concepts based on nostalgia. From the knowledge transmitted during those wonderful days on the farm, many other centres were started in England, Scotland, Canada, Mexico and the United States. For those individuals who have dedicated their lives to a life of service, the 'question' is still alive and the 'Path of Return' never ends.

6

An Introduction to Shock

When we are able to dedicate our life to a life of conscious service, we are given everything that we need for transformation to occur, not just for our fellow human beings and the planet, but also for ourselves. The passion of our inner question sets our course through life and if we can keep this 'question' alive and our intention clear, then, through our trust and the laws of synchronicity, we can begin to discover our purpose in life on earth.

Using my own life as a frame, it has been my intention to illustrate how these ideas came into play in one man's journey towards Truth. In the same way that no two experiences can be alike, the search will be different for each one of us. I have demonstrated how the world of attraction can deflect us from our aim and how we carry the patterns of the past, not just from our ancestors, but also from our 'tightening in the moment'. The chapters remaining are a distillation of the knowledge that I have been given through my experiences as it relates to healing. They are a continuation of the theme that we are all here to heal, in the recognition that the sole purpose of love is beauty.

Although it is true to say that it is the ideas that bring about change, ideas in the formative worlds remain in their embryonic state until we manifest them on earth. We are the vehicles through which Divine Order can be brought forth, but we need to keep this multi-dimensional vehicle that is called a human being in tune with the Universal Laws.

One of the most important principles in healing that has emerged from all my experiences is the idea that there is a pattern to shock. This shock can be on many different levels. If we can understand the nature of shock, we will gain valuable insight into the causes of suffering and see how patterns of behaviour, both physical and psychological, manifest in our daily lives.

My first introduction to the pattern of shock happened when I was very young. We had a favourite labrador dog that we used to enter in the championship trials but, at a certain time each year, we would have to take him completely out of the running. At an early age, he had been bitten on the nose by an adder and had gone into a coma, in which he remained for nearly a week. Every year afterwards, to the day he died at a ripe old age, at exactly the same time that the snake bite had occurred, he would go to sleep, refusing food and taking only a little water. The shock of the incident remained with him throughout his life, and being an animal, he did not know how to change that pattern.

Over the years, I began to watch myself and observe how I would automatically behave emotionally at different times of the year. I realised that this was not to do with the changing seasons alone, but that there were other, underlying causes stretching through my life. This understanding opened up new vistas and insights for me into how and why we behave. In my mid-twenties I discovered a woman teacher who was able to explain these principles and who also helped me to untangle the pattern of my own past. For over four years I studied with her so that I could be given the knowledge of how to help others to do the same thing.

Shock can also be creative, although for most people, if the word 'shock' is used, the mind immediately sees this as negative. There are shocks that can act as positive mediators at a time when we are fixed in one cycle and need to move on to another. If we could be taught this at an early age by loving parents who understood this principle, we might not get caught in the moment when the shock occurred. If we 'tighten,' on the other hand, we can fix something that is not necessarily useful, which then holds us, like flies in a honey pot, until that pattern is redeemed through the present moment.

I remember someone who, as a child, was so attached to his teddy bear that, when his brother cut it open one day, he nearly went into a comatose state. He had no memory of this event until, while in hospital for an appendectomy, he suddenly had a total recall of that time. The unknown pattern by which he had been bound was therefore recognised and released through the present moment and, as a result, his life was freed to a degree that he had not thought possible.

Moments of shock can steal a portion of our senses which then remain locked in the pattern. Until those frozen pieces of ourselves are redeemed and healed, we cannot be completely in the present moment. If we are not totally here with all of our being, we are not fully alive and thus are limited in the development of our full potential.

Human beings are not just two- or even three-dimensional. Looking out of the window into the garden or towards the mountain, we so often run into the trap of seeing only 'the view and me' or 'the mountain and me'. This is very limiting. We may 'reverse' space instead, and let the plant or the mountain see us, which will take us out of the normal world of intellectual reasoning. We can also add another dimension to the 'view' and 'the point from which we see the view' by noticing at the same time that the sun is shining. This opens us to a world of possibility. And then, beyond what we can see in any one moment is that which we can sense, and even beyond that is that which we only know exists. Can we hear at the same time as we can see, smell the scent of a beautiful rose, taste the water on our lips and feel our bodies walking along the path? We seldom make full use of these beautiful senses we have been given.

A great man once said to me, "We must love our brothers and sisters into the present moment." As we truly live in this eternal, ever present moment, other and more refined senses can be brought forth and put to use in service. One of these senses is clairvoyance. Here I am not referring to mediumship and all that that connotes, but rather addressing the literal meaning of the word, which means 'clear seeing', derived from both French and Latin roots. To see clearly means to see what actually *is* without the distortion of the limitations of the mind or false ego, often composed of opinions from the past, both from our parents and ancestors, and our judgements during this lifetime. Seeing, in the true meaning of the word, is to be able to see what is existing in the relative world and also what is invisible to the ordinary eye, in, for example, the formative worlds.

In the same way that clairvoyance is the ability to 'see' with an inner eye, clairaudience enables us to 'hear' with an inner ear. Once the concept of our own separation from the One Reality starts to loosen its tie, we are granted the ability to be in more than one place at a time. Many more inherent gifts are available to us which we can then use in conscious service for the planet and our fellow human beings, once the pattern of shock that has motivated our lives for so long has been redeemed.

7
The Pattern of Shock

If, as human beings, we aspire towards the enormous potential that lies within us, then we can begin to participate in the process of conscious evolution, rather than just in the organic evolution of our planet. Conscious evolution can only come about through conscious human beings. As we begin to tread this path of healing and discover that we are on this planet to heal, so we enter a world of life, which Gurdjieff called, 'The Experiment of Life on Earth'.

We are made up of many different, inter-penetrating subtle bodies, often called 'etheric bodies' because our composition includes fire, earth, air, water and ether. Ether is considered in physics to be an all-pervading weightless mass which is the carrying force of electro-magnetic waves. These etheric bodies are capable of carrying the electro-magnetic force to where it is needed, often through the power of directed thought. Each of these subtle bodies has its counterpart in the world that we can know with the senses, which, for the sake of definition, I have labelled a physical body, a sexual body, an emotional body, a mental-motivational body and an aspirational body, each more refined than the one before.

Although we are mainly identified with the 'physical' body, we also need to be able to observe it quite objectively, gratefully acknowledging that we have a suitable vehicle to carry us on life's journey. We can be physically handicapped and still, through understanding, be able to participate in the Divine Plan. There is no end to the possibilities lying within us. As we realise that we are continuously 'becoming' from increasingly subtle levels of vibration in the invisible worlds, so much of our fear of inadequacy can be taken away. In a sense we are all crippled in our apparent inability to *do* something about situations that seem beyond our control.

It is not difficult to understand how the physical body can undergo shock, whether it be a whiplash from a car accident, the results of an operation, or some other injury. However, a physical shock will not necessarily remain in the memory if our attitude is what we were thinking or feeling when the shock occurred. That is what fixes the pattern of the shock that can continuously affect our lives. How carefully we would walk up the stairs when we were angry or bitter if we only understood that a lost footing could 'fix' whatever we were thinking in that moment for an indefinite period of time!

The pattern of a shock is not only determined by what we were thinking or feeling at the time of the shock, but also where we were thinking from. Often we presume that thinking comes from the head, and yet the truth is that only if it were pure, unadulterated thought could this be so. Mainly our thought comes from below the belt, where fear, pride, greed, envy and resentment, all those different walls that divide us from the Truth, reside. If we could see the colour and shape of some of the things we think, and we did not have a sense of humour at the same time, it would be difficult to live with ourselves! Pure thought was described by Jesus in *The Apocryphal Acts of John:* 'I am thought, being wholly thought.'

Today there is strong agreement among the healing professions that illness stems from the mind, but it is also important to remember that the mind is made up of many levels. This is easier to understand if we return to the idea that we think and feel from different areas in the body, each area having its own special function. What we put out in thought will always come back and land in the same area where we tightened at that moment. The moment is ever-living, yet we trap it in our judgements, our fears and our illusions and thus we are not free. This does not mean to say that all negative thoughts and experiences are going to make us physically sick. If we are honest with ourselves, we could not count the number of occasions when we have had bad thoughts. It is time to say that some form of illness can manifest in the physical world as a result of a thought pattern. For example, a shock later in life can trigger off the original shock in childhood which produced a motivator in our behaviour pattern as an adult.

The physical body is material and therefore vibrates at the lowest level. Each remaining etheric body or level of vibration is more refined than the one before, although they all inter-penetrate each other and the physical as well. It is almost as though we can see them as different worlds within Unity itself, each being entirely unique and yet, in reality, not separate from the whole except through concepts of the mind.

I call the next higher level of vibration the sexual body because, for the most part, we are ruled by sexual desire. Here I am not referring to the act of sex alone, but also to the nature of desire in the first place. It is an aspect in ourselves and, if it were not there, the world would not be complete for there would be no procreation. Indeed the planet needs children, and it is love, manifesting as desire, that makes the world go round!

It is useful to notice, however, how often we are identified with our sexual body at the expense of the other bodies, and in this way, it can be dreadfully misused. The same can also be true for the physical body if it does not work in co-operation with the rest of the bodies. I fear that many who go jogging or do exercises for enlightenment's sake are merely getting further into the path of identification rather than working to free themselves from the world of illusion. Paradoxically, we do need this body as a vehicle to carry the higher forces and therefore it is important that we keep it fit so that it can function in the service of Unity. It is merely a question of how we view things. We can only be free when all the aspects of our being are in perfect balance and harmony with the life blood of the universe itself.

As a healer, many people who have been sexually abused or misused have come to me asking for help. They walk around as though they have been wounded in a war, carrying the scars with them for those who can see. I will use the following story in order to illustrate just how badly damaged the sexual body can be.

Some time ago, a young woman, twenty-seven years of age, came to me with a serious condition of the uterus. She had been advised by the medical profession that a complete hysterectomy was necessary. In reviewing her life history, it turned out that she had been raped twice, on two separate occasions, while hiking in the same area in the Rocky Mountains of Colorado. The violations were committed by two different men and two years separated the events.

Nothing happens by chance. Making inquiries, I discovered that that particular area was well known for such events. It seemed as though the area itself attracted violence. I asked whether she had ever thought about this, and whether, subconsciously, she had chosen to take that same trail after what had occurred to her two years before. The questions certainly awakened something in her but she was unable, at that time, to find any logical reason for her action. The memory was obviously too painful.

The next step was to investigate what, in herself, had brought about these rapes. It is often said that our symptom or our pain is merely our visiting card towards the understanding of our true self. Apparently, it is only by chance that a woman is raped, but, in reality, there are many factors that come into play. In all the cases I have counselled there have been subsidiary causes that have brought on the rape. Not every woman hiking in that area suffered such indignity and violence, and yet something in the area did provide a suitable environment for the men concerned. There were two factors to consider: the area itself, and the reason why one woman got into trouble and many others did not.

I discovered, with the help of the higher senses, that this woman had a considerable degree of shock in several of the etheric bodies as well as some residue in the physical body. This was not surprising. I found the main cause to be sexual shock at the age of five and a half. I questioned her deeply as to whether she had any memory of what might have occurred at that age, but try as hard as she could, she could find nothing in her memory bank connected with molestation or any related incident at that age.

Intuitively I was convinced that my findings were correct. There are techniques in healing which can be given to help a person to dream consciously and I instructed her in these, sent her home and asked her to return the next day. In the morning she came back with a look of great surprise on her face.

"You know," she said, "it was as though I was half awake and half asleep around dawn this morning. I could see quite clearly that something had indeed happened at that age, but I had never thought about it since." Her eyes were bright and she was blushing slightly. I knew that I was half way to helping her. There had already been a release of a portion of the pattern of the shock through the very act of recognition. She went on to explain that she remembered being in the shower with her elder brother, a rather large teenager, and there had been some sexual experimenting. That, in itself, would not necessarily have caused the sexual shock that I had picked up. Obviously there was more to it. I let her go on running through the memory pattern and finally said to her, "Well, did you enjoy it?" For a moment she looked as though she were five and a half years old once again. "Oh yes," she said with a deep breath, looking coy and hanging down her head.

She had tightened in that moment, felt guilty and blocked

out any memory in the conscious mind. The memory pattern, although hidden, was still there. It was that memory pattern which helped to bring on the rapes in a subconscious desire to remember the feeling she had as a child. The blocked pattern of shock also helped to manifest the physical condition in the uterus.

In this case it was not difficult to see why the young woman's disease manifested in her uterus, for it was from that area that she had been thinking at the time. Thought form, being rather like an elastic band, bounced back in its negative aspect and caused the problem. I am sure that she must also have had an inherent weakness in that area, but after the realisation that she herself had experienced in her dream, my explanation of the situation, and further counselling work that was necessary, it was not long before she was well again.

The next level of vibration I call the emotional body, or the emotional world. As in all the other worlds, there are endless dimensions to consider. Each of these different 'bodies' can contain and maintain shocks that have occurred previously, and the pattern, fixed by these shocks, can continue to affect our lives. By consciously observing within ourselves how we react to any given circumstance, we can be our own healer as we face, without blame, guilt or shame, those things that motivate our lives. Recognition is the first step in this process, in the same way that diagnosis, in the medical profession, is the first step towards the recovery of the patient.

Just as we can become attached to the sexual world, so we can be totally identified with the emotional world. Without feeling, without the deeper emotions, we would not be complete human beings and yet it is important to recognise that there are also many negative emotions. The emotional world is given to us to use rather than allowing ourselves to be used by the emotional world. Our aim, after all, is to become conscious human beings, not identified with or attached to the different worlds, but instead, glorifying in the totality of life, not coldly, but passionately with the meaning of it all.

I remember a classical case of emotional shock that occurred to me in southern Turkey.★ I was studying in a residential setting with my spiritual teacher at that time. The night before the incident, there had been a gypsy wedding to which the whole village was invited to attend. Preparations had been going on for days, special awnings had been set up over the courtyard in the cafe, coloured lights were brought in and all about was an air of tremendous festivity. It was unusual for such an event to take place, for the gypsies lived far out on the plains of Anatolia and seldom came into the town, except occasionally to sell their wares.

When the wedding took place, people were climbing on the roofs to get a good look while others were up in the trees. After the sun went down, the dancing began, the wine, the raki and the beer flowed and the gypsy band played with such fervour that it was impossible for me not to dance. And dance I did until nearly dawn. My teacher, who, up until then, had said nothing, finally expressed his disgust at my 'performance'. By then the sky had turned black and ominous, and there was a certain pressure in the air. Most of the people had returned to their homes and there were just a few left cleaning up.

That same night, after a brief sleep, I was awakened by the sound of a huge storm with lightning, hail and high winds. It was still dark and I lay awake, afraid to go to sleep for fear I would miss the pre-arranged meeting with my teacher soon after dawn. The storm itself did not last very long. When it stopped, I noticed how the pressure in the air had changed. There was also a strange sensation everywhere which made me almost afraid to get ready for the meeting.

The first light then appeared, signifying that the sun

★*The Last Barrier*, Reshad Feild, Element Books.

would soon break through. As it got lighter, I managed to struggle out of bed. Opening the blinds, I looked out on to the courtyard of the house. In the courtyard and on the roofs of the houses I saw nothing but millions and millions of tiny toads. It was like a moving river of toads, so thick that I could scarcely see the road. At first I thought that I had gone completely mad and sat down on the bed again, checking to see if I was still in my body. "This can't be true," I said to myself hopefully, but it was true when I looked out once more. By then the sun was up and I needed to move quickly if I was to be on time for my appointment on the beach with my teacher. I still had not washed and I was completely overwhelmed. My emotional body rumbled with the shock. If anyone had tightened in the moment, I had!

Finally I plucked up courage, washed, dressed and went down the stairs to the patio where I gingerly tried to pick my way through the throng without hurting any of them. I was like a ballet dancer on the points of his shoes. I walked out across the village square until I came to a path that led to the beach. Where had all these baby toads come from? Did they come from the lightning storm and drop from the clouds? I certainly was in no collected state,★ one of the conditions for the impending meeting. I knew that my teacher would be waiting for me, toads or no toads. As I walked, a dim memory came out of the past. Had there not been a plague of toads mentioned in the Bible? Could this be a punishment given out by God?

My teacher was there, sitting outside the deserted café, his walking stick in front of him. I suspect I looked very sheepish since he made no comment. The beach also was covered with toads. I sat down, doing everything that I could to be in a collected state. "What's wrong?" he questioned. "You are shaking. What for? Didn't you do your clearing exercise† last night, or were you not together enough in your senses to remember?"

★See page 120
†See page 112

At first I felt extremely ashamed and also very frightened, but to this day, I am still grateful to him, for during our meeting he helped me to unwind the tightening within my emotional body. If he had not, that experience could have stayed in my mind, causing so much fear and guilt that my entire life could have been affected. There *were* toads... They were not illusions of the mind. Even my teacher agreed that there were toads although we just continued with our work as though nothing unusual had happened. Identification was not allowed, no matter how difficult it was to remain awake during certain situations. To make it even more bizarre, when the sun became too hot and we started to walk back along the beach to the square, and then to the house, the toads had disappeared as miraculously as they had appeared. Thus, the shock turned into a miracle rather than a disease, leaving me with a sense of wonder and awe as to how these things can happen.

It is important to understand that these subtle bodies or worlds are not 'higher' or 'lower' in relationship to each other. That is a concept of the mind. As I have already mentioned, they are inter-penetrating, different rates of vibration. There are even Higher Worlds but they are un-manifested worlds, waiting to be received into our world when we have sufficiently prepared our vehicles, on all levels, to receive them.

The next world I term the mental-motivational world. Consider the idea of motive and intention and how, if our motive is pure, things can manifest in the relative world for the good of mankind. Just as all the other bodies can be in a state of shock, and as such, harmed, so can the mental-motivational body. By this stage, though, it is unlikely that the mental-motivational body can be harmed through shock, without the emotional, sexual and therefore, in turn, the physical body being affected. In the understanding that each world is a carrying force for the one 'above' it, the more subtle the vibration, the more effect there is right down into the physical. The following story relates to the mental–motivational body:

Not long ago a dear friend made a mistake when driving his car. While he was attempting to alter the station on his radio, he inadvertently hit the soft shoulder of the road. The car went out of control and turned over three times down a cliff. As all this was happening, he remembered a breathing practice* to help him remain as conscious as possible. When the car, then a total wreck, came to a halt, he found himself in the back seat without even a scratch. If, on the other hand, he had tightened in the moment, he would have almost certainly been seriously hurt or killed, and whatever he was thinking at the time would have remained locked in the moment, affecting the different levels of his being. The reason that I include this story relative to the mental–motivational body is that, after a long discussion, he explained to me that his motives for driving the car at that precise time and in that direction were not at all clear.

The road that leads to the Truth is steep and, at times, precipitous. Indeed it does require tremendous patience and perseverance to keep on going when it seems that all odds are against us, when there is nothing left to hold on to except that inner cry, that burning question as to why we exist at all. The further on we go in the work of transformation, the more important it is to continue with whatever practices we are given. They provide us with the necessary balance and co-operation in the different worlds, which, along with a clear intention, enable us to proceed safely on our journey.

Still in the light of the mental–motivational body, a similar situation happened to me. I had been invited to meet a woman who was very advanced in the healing and 'esoteric' fields. She had been initiated into some of the highest levels and perhaps, although my motive was clear, my timing was off because of a lurking ambition, somewhere along the

*See page 109

line, to discover what she knew. Remember, there are many levels in each of these worlds.

A friend offered to drive me that Sunday from Scotland to London, where the meeting was to take place. The necessary arrangements had been made. As the meeting was an important one, I was determined to get there on time, even though it was a long, eight to ten hour drive. We left late, which wasn't a good sign. Often things can go wrong if we decide upon a time and then break our own word to ourselves.

Just before we crossed the border between Scotland and England, my friend decided to accelerate from about 70 m.p.h. to nearly 80 m.p.h. on a wet road whilst manoeuvring a sharp right hand turn. The skid seemingly went on forever before we plunged over the edge of the road. We crashed into a tree, and then bounced on down, rolling and turning, before finally being brought to a halt by a thick steel fence. I suspect we all have some sort of private prayer we use in emergencies, and I remember very well, as we went into the skid, repeating the Jesus prayer continuously on the breath and in the heart. By the time we went over the edge, I was completely conscious and awake, in the present moment, and ready for what seemed inevitable. Unaccountably no one was hurt except my dog, who went into a panic, bumping his nose on the windscreen as he was flung from the back seat. If I had not known of these different worlds and had instead tightened, we might have been seriously injured. The other, finer levels of vibration as well could have been locked in the moment.

We crawled out of the car, looking back up to the road which now seemed far above us. As is almost inevitable, it was not long before a car drew up and a nice Scottish couple, out for a Sunday drive, looked down and, after having asked us if we were all right, said, "Now, would you like a cup of tea?" Perhaps the very incongruity of it all helped to release any shock that might have occurred.

Thus far we have looked at shock at the physical level and in three of the etheric bodies, manifested as sexual shock, emotional shock and mental-motivational shock. Shock, acting as a wound, helps to produce blocks in our lives which then may cause us to over-compensate. In any given situation, the effect of a shock, on whatever level, may manifest itself down into the physical world. I have a firm conviction that cancer is the manifestation in the physical body of the chaos that is held in the other, subtle bodies. It is from where we think, as well as what we think, that has a deep effect on the results of negative thoughts.

In no way am I saying that the knowledge of working with shock patterns is a panacea for all illness. Rather, in the same way that this knowledge was awakened in me, I am hoping to awaken in others the basic and yet seldom taught principles of shock, so that we can see a little deeper into our responsibility in being born, having children and being custodians of our planet.

If there is damage to our 'aspirational' body, we lose that instrument with which we aspire. So many people are raised in expectation by their parents, little realising that expectation, as it forms itself in the etheric field, damages the aspirational body, sometimes so badly that the child never recovers that inner vision which can lead him on to better things. Perhaps one of the greatest sins, if there is such a thing as sin, is for a parent to bring up a child in expectation. In reality, when this occurs, it is the parents who are attempting to cover up their own failures and, by trying to hide behind their children, they do them immense harm. The 'aspirational' body is the highest rate of vibration, and therefore the most difficult to heal.

Let me give an example of how this damage can be done. Imagine a little girl, the jewel of her father's eye, who is spoiled by her parents before she has hardly grown up. Spoiling a child is almost as bad as child abuse, for, in later life, it lowers the dignity of that human being to a degree that is often painful to observe. This little girl, whom I shall call Annie, had been promised a pony on her fifth birthday. She was thrilled, excited and spent many hours with her parents looking at picture books of ponies and horses, to such an extent that she was dreaming of horses each night. Her whole life revolved around the thought of her fifth birthday. There was a little paddock behind the house and she and her father spent many hours tending it, and building a fence around it for the day the pony would arrive.

Annie told all her friends about the coming event and invited them to come to her birthday party to meet the pony she had heard about for so long. She was so overwhelmed that she did not even notice that her parents were going through a very difficult time in their relationship, and that when she went to bed, they were shouting and fighting with each other. Sound fixes pattern and therefore, even in her sleep, the effects of the arguments were beginning to tell in the child's electro-magnetic field.

The day before Annie's birthday her father went to work as usual, but he did not return home before she went to bed. Her mother told her that he had to work late at the office and assured her that she was not to worry. Dawn came, and Annie woke up early. Perhaps the pony had already arrived and that was the reason her father had been late the night before. Looking out of the window, she saw the paddock was empty. She then went downstairs and crept into her parents' room. After all, it was her birthday! Her mother was still sleeping, but her father was not there. She panicked, went totally into despair, and when her mother woke, she cried so much that she had to be given a warm, chocolate drink to calm her down. It was then that she was told her father was not coming back. He had gone away, and there was no pony.

The shock of that event is easily understood. Annie had aspired towards that day, her birthday, and the arrival of the pony she had been promised for so long. The shock, on at least three of the subtle levels, became established before she was seven years of age. Although the memory of the bitter disappointment eventually wore off, when she was a teenager she had a bitter resentment for men. She would taunt them sexually and then laugh at them. She married in her early twenties, became pregnant almost at once, and when the child was only about a year old, she left both her husband and the child and landed up on heavy drugs.

Let us review the sequence of events. Annie had been brought up in expectation, spoiled as a young child, and was then bitterly disappointed at the age of five, all for the sake of a pony. She was blocked at that point in time by the shock, and was finally left with nothing to aspire to, and little or no sense of responsibility. It took a long time to help her face the memory pattern of that event so that she could start her life anew.

Sound fixes pattern. The sound we make in front of our children, and the children around us, has a direct bearing on the moment and thus, our responsibility as adults is enormous. We need to be careful what we think and what we say, for even a thought has a sound. Surely we aspire to make this world a more healthy place in which to live, for our children and our children's children.

8

Breathing Alive

Many books have been written on the subject of breath, particularly in the Yoga tradition, but remarkably little material can be found in the western world, for the western mentality. In considering breath, I first want to stress the word 'service'. There is so much pain and suffering in the world. Often within ourselves it is hard to sit down and complete a practice, such as a breathing practice, towards the healing of the world, when perhaps we are in great pain ourselves. The paradox is that often when we do remember that we are here to heal, things ease up for us in our own lives and we are offered a flash of what our purpose may be.

Most of the time we are asleep and we presume many things, not the least of which is breath itself. Breath is Life! If we contemplate these three words alone, we can understand our responsibility in being conscious of our breath and also gain encouragement in learning how to breathe under all circumstances. In our contemplation we can say *breath* is life, breath *is* life, or breath is *life,* each emphasising a different aspect of breath to be discovered. In order to be truly awake we need to understand the importance of breath. We can, for example, follow the breath through the nostrils and watch its circulation in the body. We can see its transforming effect on the cells and molecules, and know that it can be a carrying force of healing energy to those parts of the body that need it. Our breath is not just limited to our own body but can be transmitted across time and space. We can also learn how to breathe for another person when the going gets rough.

Breath is the key to conscious birth, sex and death.

Consider the man who stands by his wife through labour and at the moment of birth, keeping the strength and rhythm of his breath constant so that it is easier for her to relax. Conscious breathing is also vital in the sexual act, which can be the most sacred on earth if we wish to consciously participate in the Divine Order. And, at the moment of death, even if the person who is going to pass is unconscious, by breathing consciously, using the Mother's breath*, there can be deep peace in the room.

Obviously all this needs a certain degree of practice. Unfortunately few of us were taught such things at school or in our homes, but it is never too late to learn! The great key towards learning the art of breathing is not to expect, however subtly, any reward from the practice. The mind is ambitious, but we must remember that we are here to heal and be healed, not to gain power and favours for ourselves.

Let us look at a typical day, beginning with the moment we wake up, and observe the implications of breath. Perhaps we yawn or stretch a little until we are ready to get out of bed and begin our day. When we are lying horizontally, our breath is not the same as when we are sitting or standing. Both positions bring in different aspects of energy. When we are lying down, we have a certain type of magnetism, essentially related to the time of day when the sun sets and we begin our night-time journey towards sleep. Equally, when we rise from bed into a vertical position, we have an energy of a different order, necessary to complete our work during the day. In the same way, if we breathe consciously while lying on our right side, we find a different sensation to breathing while facing the left. That is why it is said that if we are unable to pray standing, sitting or on our knees, then we should pray lying on our right side. The quality of the breath is more receptive in this position.

If we are absolutely awake and conscious as we get out of bed, we are able to blend in breath, the word and the sound

*See page 109

of the different aspects of night and day. The first practice in the morning is to decide to get out of bed, as opposed to just haphazardly rolling out and drifting aimlessly into the day. We consciously get up, being awake to the exact moment that our feet touch the ground. The bed will surely wait for us for another night! Sitting on the edge of the bed, we then offer ourselves to the beginning of the new day, saying within, "May I be allowed to be of service this day?" At this time we also say the prayer of our choice before we stand up, and then, remembering the breath, we move into the next step of our lives. It is amazing how helpful this is.

The morning proceeds. We eat breakfast and then go to work. If we watch carefully as we move through the day, our breath starts to change. It is as though we have built-in gear shifts in the tides of our breathing which alter according to what is apparently going on in the moment.

Let us say, for example, that we get into our car, drive towards our place of work, and suddenly find ourselves in a traffic jam. Imagine that we left a little late from home, which increased the rhythm of our breath, and now, from the fear of being late, we start to develop anger and frustration because things are not going the way we had hoped they would. The breath, accelerating from our fear of being late, gets stifled in anger. In both these states, we could not be true agents for healing. In the first instance, we would not be in the present moment through speeding along in hope, and in the latter case, we would also not be in the present moment, through the stifling of our breath. If we then lost our temper and shouted at the other drivers, we certainly could not call ourselves healers and we might even cause an accident. True healing can only occur in the present moment.

The same is true in our emotional lives. If we are on top of the breath, then our consciousness is not submerged by our emotions. However, most of us get it backwards. What consciousness we have is totally immersed in a sea of emotional turmoil.

There is hope! Through learning, first of all, why it is useful to breathe, and then learning how to breathe, we can once again get on top of the breath. The higher aspects of our being, interconnected as they are with the Higher Worlds themselves, can then work through us, carried on the wind of change that blows through a conscious man or woman. This is the necessary change from stagnation, illness and negative emotions. It is a great challenge.

We all make mistakes, otherwise we would never learn. Let us say, for the sake of this analogy, that we continued to forget about breath and healing during the day. We arrived late at the office and stormed through the door. We found that there was a new secretary, and the letters were misplaced that we were meant to write. The coffee was cold and then, just as we were making a fresh brew, the power went off. At this point, about the only thing that could save the disastrous day would be the remembrance of the sacredness of breath. If we worked with the Mother's breath*, the office would calm down and order would prevail once again.

Breath – conscious breathing – has a direct relationship to time. Our experience of time completely alters if we are on top of the breath. If we had left home at the time we decided we would, having said goodbye to our husband, wife, children or friends for the day, stopped for a moment to collect ourselves, smiled as we got into the car, and *decided* to drive consciously to the office, then perhaps there would have been no traffic jam. If we had left on time, we might have gone straight through all the other drivers who had not made their own decisions and therefore, were still caught in the traffic jam!

*See page 109

The day continues at the office. Just as each hour is different and has its own feeling, so does each day. What we do on a Monday, which is influenced by the moon, we would not do on a Tuesday, influenced by Mars, or on a Thursday, influenced by Jupiter. Each day has its own quality. In the same way that planting at certain cycles of the moon increases the chances of the plants being healthy and strong, so, by planning our activities in conjunction with the particular quality of each hour during the day, we can establish order and balance in our own lives.

If we watch the breath during the day, we will find that approximately every hour there is a subtle change, not just in the rhythm but also in the positioning of the breath. These changes happen automatically although we seldom notice them at the time. Usually there is more 'vibration' or energy going through one nostril than the other. If we are aware of our breathing, we may, at one moment, be able to sense the breath more easily through the right nostril and then again, at another moment, through the left. When we feel more energy going through the right nostril then we are in a position of being more positive and it is a good time to take action. Equally, when the sensation of breath is in the left nostril, we will be more receptive. If the breath is equal on both sides, we have a balance between the active and the passive.

We can change our breathing from one nostril to the other as the need arises. If it is necessary to attend a meeting in a positive manner, then, in the space of about three minutes, we can change our breath to pass through the right nostril. If we are ready to receive what we need to hear in any one moment, then it is important to have the correct vibratory rate going through the left nostril. It is much more difficult to get into the totally balanced breath but with visualisation and practice, we can learn to breathe through the membrane that separates the right and left nostrils.

The more we work with conscious breathing, the more we will be able to live in harmony in a chaotic world. We will find that we identify less and less with situations and thus can stand above the grinding clash of opposites in the bank or supermarket. Gradually we begin to build in an inner observer that is more sensitive to the moment and so we are able to see what is needed at any one time and also know how we can best help.

If we are sitting in a room with a group of people, we are all apparently breathing in the same air and breathing out the distilled air after it has passed through our systems. Yet there is also a way of choosing the air we breathe, although only by making the experiment ourselves can this be shown to be true. It is well worth the trouble taken. The key is to choose the finest *quality* of air that we can. This is done with what is sometimes called 'Creative Imagination'. It is not fantasy, but rather an inner gift which can be brought forth as a creative act.

A question might arise as to how we can choose the finest quality of air in a room full of smokers. The answer is that it is difficult but still possible through visualisation. By judging the smokers or the smoke, we become identified with the situation. If it is vitally necessary for us to attend a particular function, the presence or absence of smoke should not be our sole deterrent. Our aim, remember, is to be able to breathe under all conditions.

We can imagine that we are standing by an ocean or by a beautiful stream or pure mountain water and, holding this picture, continue to breathe with the Mother's breath*, the 7 – 1 – 7 – 1 – 7 rhythm. It is also possible to breathe from a particular star or planet for balance. If we need extra male strength, we can breathe from Mars, which will increase the element of iron in our bodies. If we need to be more receptive, we can alternatively breathe while visualising the planet Venus, increasing the element of copper within us.

*See page 109

We can even visualise the sacred places on the planet, which are of so much benefit to the world, as we breathe. We might imagine the places in the Himalayas where the holy men assemble, or cities like Jerusalem, Chartres in France, Glastonbury in England or the huge medicine wheel in Wyoming. It is all done with breath and visualisation and the gift is ours.

Let us return to our imaginary day. If we eat consciously during the lunch break, respectfully watching the breath, we will have all the energy that is needed for the afternoon. Our attitude towards food in healing should be the same as that in breath. It is important that we do not take anything for granted in our lives and that we remember to be grateful. We can then share this deep sense of gratitude with others who might have forgotten it.

The afternoon can be a sleepy and difficult time to concentrate. Once again, if we use the breath consciously, we can make things much easier. Each breath may be our last. We never know. We come into this world on the breath and we go out of this world on the breath. If life seems difficult, during the afternoon or at any other time, we can always sit down for a moment and contemplate this.

Soon it will be time to leave the office, get back into the car, and face the journey home and the fumes, the frustrated human beings, the blaring radios and the toll gates. It all seems to take so much time. How do we manage to deal with such situations day after day without getting an ulcer or high blood pressure? Many people put themselves into a totally numbed state, which is one solution, but it is not a conscious way. It is merely a method of being totally unconscious so that the discomfort need not be faced.

If we are on top of the breath, then we live in the ever-present moment and that is what a healer is here for. As I have said, we are all healers in our own way. We must be conscious and awake. We need to be present at every breath we take. Freedom lies at the exact point between the in-breath and the out-breath and at that moment, grace may enter. We never know when this might happen. It could happen on the motorway. The traffic jam may be an excellent time to practise the art of breathing, so that by the time we arrive home, we will be completely ready to greet our friends or family. We will not be carrying all the weight of the day on our shoulders and bringing it into the house. Instead, we will be free to be of service from the moment we cross the threshold.

Once we are home, we will probably want to take a bath or shower to wash away the dirt of the day. Here is another opportunity to use the breath. As we bathe, we can consciously breathe in the moisture. Breath carries moisture. Water, on the other hand, is a conductor of electricity, and thought-forms are electrical impulses. By being conscious of the breath and the moisture in the shower, we can purify our subtle bodies, where thought-forms of the subtlest nature may have attached themselves to us without our noticing them.

Now we are ready for the evening and all that that may bring. We have worked hard to keep on top of the breath and on top of time. For the completion of the day, we make our decision exercise* and finally do the clearing exercise†. We can then sleep at peace, ready for what the next day will bring.

Breath is Life! We breathe in only to breathe out and thus we learn to balance the in-breath with the out-breath. We watch the breath and see how it enters us, and how it can be used for good. We visualise as we breathe. We breathe for others in times of stress. Through visualisation and breath, we gather the beauty and energy we need in order to be of service. As Ibn al' Arabi, a great Sufi mystic, once said, 'All is contained in the Divine Breath, like the day in the morning's dawn.'

*See page 115
†See page 112

9

Permission and Authority in the Healing Profession

The question of 'Permission and Authority' in the healing profession is a matter that concerns us all, in whatever field we work. It is something that seldom, if ever, comes up in the various trainings that we are given. The further we go into the realm of thought and prayer the less we are taught the fact that we need to have the *permission* of the person or group for whom we pray. We need to question very deeply whether we have the necessary *authority* (and here we imply a fine degree of knowledge) to, as it were, launch thought-forms into the ether, which most surely will try to manifest themselves somewhere or other.

I often tell the story of a time when I was living in Los Angeles and running an intensive school of transformation. All was going well until, for no apparent reason, I began to feel ill at ease. I felt as though I was sinking deeper and deeper into the mire with an enormous loss of energy. I sat down and meditated on this and the answer was given to me. A large group of people had felt that I needed to be prayed for during that period. When I realised what was going on, I immediately telephoned them, thanked them very much for their concern and asked them to please stop their prayers. Shortly I started to regain my energy and to feel better. Later I was able to travel to the group and explain that what they were doing, despite their goodwill, was to project their group and individual *concepts* of what they thought that I needed. It is a common occurrence for people to mistake their opinions for real prayer.

The question arises, then, how can we *know* for certain that we have permission, and have the necessary knowledge and authority to act? In the medical profession it is the patient who first comes and asks for help, and then the doctor does his or her best to remedy the pain and suffering. Permission is granted by the patient for the treatment. If there is to be an operation in the hospital, the patient is required to sign a form relinquishing the doctor of the responsibility for the operation, since there can never be any promises made. The patient takes on the responsibility of handing over his or her body to the operating table. Is it not a similar situation when we are dealing with the realms of the mind and the causal worlds? How often do we ask within whether we have the right to assist in the process of change through our own strength, mind and thought-forms? There are times when it may be necessary that the person we so want to help remain ill for a while in order that a certain lesson can be learned or some dross burnt out.

We do have a protection in all these matters if we ask the three questions that I stress to those who study the methods of healing I use and teach. The three questions are: 'May I?' 'Should I?' and 'Can I?' The implications that lie within them are far reaching and it is advisable that people look deeply into the nature of the questions. Remember that these rules or laws do not just apply to members of the healing profession but can also be used in any decision-making activity.

We are all interconnected by invisible threads. There is a right time and place for everything under the sun. As men and women, it is our direct responsibility to mark well the formula of our days and not do anything without careful thought. I often quote the poet, Francis Thompson 'Thou canst not stir a flower without troubling of a star.' If we are truly honest within ourselves these questions can help us know whether we have the necessary authority and the right permissions to work with or for a patient, or to work with the land and the planet itself. If only the land developers would ask the three questions before erecting yet another bunch of houses in the wrong place!

The meaning of 'May I?' on the surface is easy to comprehend. It is asking *permission* to do whatever is deemed necessary in the present moment. It is like saying over the phone to a friend, "May I come over today?" In the first place it is a question of manners and then there are deeper levels of meaning. Suppose, for example, we ask this question, without asking it with all the passion that we can muster within, and the person on the other end of the telephone says, "No!" We might even fall into resentment and thus the question backfires. Whenever we ask a question we need to ask it with *all* of our being and then the right answer will come for all those involved. It is almost as though we need to be so finely tuned, like a musical instrument, that what lies behind the question can be heard correctly, and the reply comprehended.

In this first question we are asking permission from the Highest as well as the individual, or group, concerned. Through this question, through this connection, the High Self can bring the answer into the relative world, and then we can proceed. It is important not to proceed without this permission.

The second question, 'Should I?' can best be understood by including the nature of *time*. As I said before, there is a right time for everything. When we really ask this question in all sincerity we will understand that time is of the utmost importance in any form of healing. I know that this sounds obvious but the art of asking a question is seldom taught at school. If we contemplate this, perhaps we can come to understand a little about time itself. 'Should I?' brings us into permission *in time,* just as 'May I?' is asking permission from a Source which is outside time.

The last question, 'Can I?' implies that there is a state in which we are at any one moment. Perhaps we are simply not capable of helping on that day or at that moment of time. Perhaps we are not well, too low on energy, or not in a suitably collected state. Perhaps that which we are asked to heal is not in a state of readiness.

'Can I?' is just as big a question as the first two. I recollect a patient coming to me who had had trouble sleeping for nearly five years. She had been incorrectly diagnosed for a back injury and had received various treatments over the years, all of which had done her more harm than good. I asked the three questions for permission to do what I could and received affirmatives on each of them. She then slept for seven nights in a row. Naturally I was very happy for her, but, a week later, she called me and said that she wanted nothing further to do with me. I was surprised, to say the least, and reviewed my questions. Had I asked them correctly? In this case I had. The woman wanted to continue drawing false attention to herself and so there was nothing further for me to do. Nonetheless, because of the apparent failure, I undertook a lot of soul-searching. Maybe at that time I was an instrument to bring her to question why she continued to seek help from all these different people when in fact she could be a healer for herself.

I am using these stories to illustrate the possibilities that lie inherent within all of us. Whenever I remember these events, I am reminded again and again of our responsibility in being born human and thus potentially healers.

One day I was telephoned by a woman who said that her husband was desperately ill. He was in his late seventies. I asked them both to come for an interview with me. During our conversation, it was singularly obvious that the cancer had taken such hold on him that, according to both orthodox and unorthodox methods of healing, there was little that could be done. Having considered the three questions, I told them I would do everything I could in the given circumstances. The man was in terminal pain. His wife was very busy tending to all the details. The most important thing I was able to do at that time was to establish a deep inner connection with him on the soul level, which helped to remove his fear and tension in facing death.

For a few days I did not hear from them and then I received

another telephone call from the wife. She said that her husband had asked to come and see me again. He arrived, frail and weak, and my wife and I went to help him out of the car. Bringing him inside, we all sat together and shared tea. After a while, when things had settled, he said, "I have come to say goodbye." We held hands for a moment. His wife was calm and there was peace in the room. I can still remember his face. It was a face that had accepted life and death as one. The next day his wife telephoned to tell us that he had died in peace without any pain.

Are we not here to heal? What had I done? I had given him the knowledge that is so vital and important in our lives, the knowledge that he was loved.

I would like to finish with a story about a woman who was in difficult emotional straits. She was married, with children, and had little extra money available. One day, a rather wealthy friend turned up on her doorstep, saying that she had had 'guidance' to give money to the woman who, she felt, needed the help of a suitable counsellor. That sounded fine, initially, and the woman in despair commenced the highly expensive therapy. However, she soon decided that she did not like the counsellor and consequently gave up the treatment. Her friend became bitter because, it turned out, the counsellor was her own therapist. A letter then came saying that the money had only been a loan, and the husband was blamed for not being able to pay back the rather large sum that was apparently 'given' but actually lent. If only the three questons had been asked. Goodwill is not enough as is illustrated in the proverb: 'The road to Hell is paved with good intentions.'

10

Healing the Land

If the purpose of life on earth is towards the conscious evolution of both mankind and the planet itself, then we must not forget that just as we need to heal and be healed, so the planet requires conscious human beings to redeem the unnecessary suffering it has witnessed. We are often afraid of increasing our sensitivity because of the inner pain we feel when we suddenly realise the harm that has been done. Yet, now is the time when we simply have to wake up to our responsibility. It is easy to avoid the issues by saying that it is a superhuman job to clean up the wastage, the pollution and the appalling things we have done to our cities, mountains, rivers, streams and even the oceans themselves. I am certain, however, that given sufficient knowledge and an open heart, we can find ways to help.

Today we have only to look out of our windows to see the chaos we have perpetrated. Look at the telephone poles with their sagging wires, criss-crossing with no order at all, and at the electricity pylons and power lines. It has now been proved scientifically that these structures create an electro-magnetic field that affects the will and the psyche of a human being, not to mention the rest of God's kingdoms. Are we willing to bring order out of chaos?

Perhaps it has taken all the devastation that we see and hear of to begin to awaken people to the fact that we are custodians of our planet, as we are custodians of the land we apparently 'own' and the property in which we live. We are the custodians in this fleeting life. We cannot take the land with us when we die, but we can do a good job in keeping it going for our children and our children's children.

We often forget the interconnectedness of all life, and the fact that, like a hologram, our home and the land we live on is part and parcel of, and representative of, the whole. Beauty is contagious as love is contagious. The care that we give towards manifesting God's beauty in our gardens will not go unnoticed. Maybe the sight of a daffodil or a rose bud in our garden will awaken in our neighbours what they once knew but have forgotten and then they too will be inspired to make a garden of their own. In this way, an entire village can be healed, for not only is there harmony on the land, with roses blooming, herbaceous borders bursting with colour and fresh vegetables waiting to be picked, but also there is harmony in the souls of those who work on the land. The earth gives back to us a hundredfold all the attention that we give to her.

We can learn from what has been useful in the past. Take for example, the stately homes of Europe, where beauty has manifested on a grand scale. These homes were constructed according to sacred proportions, in a place commanding a view; the landscape gardener worked in partnership with the architect and the builders so that each aspect of the estate blended together, with little or no separation. Flower and vegetable borders were laid out in certain geometric forms to produce a 'sound' of harmony. Sitting in a sunken rose garden of a seventeenth century estate, watching the birds, the butterflies and the bees, who would not be filled with an awe of God's beauty? In China, this respect for order and balance was transmitted through the ancient art of Feng Shui, which was based on the relationship between the land, the buildings constructed and the human psyche. In England, this knowledge, also known as Geomancy, has been carried through the Celtic and Druid traditions, whereas in America, the American Indians, in their understanding, have been guardians of the land.

Throughout my life, I have been granted opportunities to learn about healing the land. Having been brought up in the beauty of the English countryside, I gained an inner sense of harmony at an early age. As I have said I was first introduced to the lore or laws of the land under the supervision of the gardener, the gamekeeper and his wife, and our cook, all who worked on the family estate. These principles were then added to, at a later time, by my work with the Druids.

There is little that can be read about the Druids, except the exterior form, because their inner secrets have been hidden from the prying eyes of those who would not know what to do with such sacred knowledge. The Druids know an enormous amount about beauty and harmony and what is required to keep them in proportion. They understand the invisible web of energy that is everywhere and they work with the ley lines in the invisible electro-magnetic lines of force that surround the earth. Ley lines were originally used in a certain way to produce flow and power at places such as Stonehenge. For the same reason, all the stately homes were built on them. Sacred buildings, such as churches and cathedrals, were often erected at the intersection of three ley lines. Today the knowledge of the Druids is coming back again although it is not taken for granted so much now as it has been for the past one hundred and fifty years.

The Druid initiates used to take me with them and point out which structures had been built on the correct place and which ones had not. They explained how, in one house, the people were happy and had children who would grow up smiling, while in another house there was anger, bitterness, resentment and fear. They begged me and others not to presume but to understand so that we could be more of service. Sometimes they would put rocks in certain places in the countryside which, they said, would help balance the environment. At other times, they would recommend replanting trees where they had been cut down. "After all," they would say, "we do have to have chlorophyl in our atmosphere, don't we?"

On certain days in the year, particularly the solstices, the Druids gather in a sacred spot to perform the rituals that have gone on for thousands of years. When I first came to America, I noted that some of the Indian ceremonies were remarkably similar. It is said that the Druids did come to America, as did the Celts, as early as 2000 to 1400 BC, but that the knowledge they brought was mainly lost. True knowledge never dies, however, although it can be swept under the glamour of the rug or carpet. Sooner or later, the rug will fade and when it is taken up, the knowledge will still be there for those who are truly interested.

The earth revealed even more of her secrets to me when I was a navigating officer in the navy. On a calm night, it was awe-inspiring, when taking bearings, to notice the billions of stars in their correct patterns. I realised then, that each planet and perhaps each star had its influence upon us, just as the moon draws the tides and the sun gives life to the earth. It was impossible for me to take life for granted.

I resolved to learn all I could about how to restore order where there is pain and suffering and how to redeem the greed of man, when he builds structures in the wrong places that adversely affect the surrounding area. The more I considered all this, the more I felt myself being drawn to certain people who held this knowledge. During this period, I found that I had the natural gift of water divining, and managed to apply the art to many related matters. A dowser does not work just with water, but is able to find many things. He may, for example, measure the proportions that are most harmonious for a particular building and then determine its relationship to the natural shape and contours of the land.

One of the people I met was an initiate of the Zoroastrian religion. From an early age he had understood the magic of natural order and he was a superb diviner. As part of his profession he practised an art, which I call 'Acupuncture of the Land'. This is the art of harnessing the natural flow lines, or ley lines, for certain purposes. With his methods, he was able to mend a break in a ley line or to correct a negative vortex of energy.

The land has memory and therefore every act of violence is registered on Mother Earth. We all know that strange sense we have when we go somewhere and something is not right. Strip mining always produces a tingling sensation in my solar plexus and a longing to get out of the area as fast as possible. Another example can be seen in Glencoe, in the Highlands of Scotland, where a famous massacre took place. Although one has to drive through the glen to get to the western Highlands and the Hebrides, few people ever stop. Some say that they hear the sounds of the massacre, the guns and the clashing of steel, and that they can sense the smell of blood.

There are meridians in and around the planet that work in a similar way to those in the human body. If there is disharmony due to an illness or lack of flow, an acupuncturist does his or her best to correct the points and free the blocked energy for the person. Many extraordinary cures have been made in this field. In the same way that an acupuncturist can help in this manner, so a geomancer can aid in bringing back harmony to the land by redeeming the long-lasting effects of man's mistakes.

There are various methods that a geomancer works with. Unlike the tiny needles used in traditional acupuncture, I use eighteen inch iron rods with copper sleeves which are driven into the ground at a specific spot and for a certain reason. Iron represents Mars, a masculine principle, while copper is the metal of Venus, which is feminine. Thus, there is a beautiful blend of male and female, yin and yang, positive and negative.

I would like to illustrate a few cases of geomancy, the science of earth energies, in which I have been involved.

In the first case a young couple, happily married with a small child, lived in England in what had once been one of the workmen's cottages on the estate of the man's father, a well-known peer of the realm. The main house on the property had been built in the mid-seventeenth century and had been lived in by their family for many generations. There had always been a sense of security, peace and harmony of which everyone was aware. Then something suddenly came about to change it all.

In geomancy, we look to the signs to give us the information we need in order to help. In this case, for no apparent reason, the family's cooker burst into flames one day. The cooker in question is well known in England. It is thoroughly reliable, burns only solid fuel and simply does not burst into flames! The young couple were devastated, since they lost most of their fine kitchen ware in the fire.

For a time things settled down but the couple said that they were becoming increasingly aware of a certain tension between them, a sense of 'suspicion', they told me. Soon afterwards, the next shock occurred. They were staying with friends for the weekend and when they returned to their own house, they found that it had been flooded. Again they lost many of their treasured belongings, and it was almost too much for them to bear. The plumber who was called in informed them that there were no broken pipes and that the main water pipe was unharmed. They then called in the local authority and the water board, who, after prodding and poking, announced that there had been an underground river flowing nearby, which had suddenly broken away from its normal water table and caused the flooding. The resolution was to make a cut into the land to drain away the water. This was done, the mud cleared out, the furniture restored and once more things returned to normal. Or had they? By this time the couple was having continuous fights and the child was constantly crying and kept having coughs and colds. It was a miserable spectacle.

One day, through a mutual contact, the couple heard about the type of work a geomancer does, and they contacted me in London. I asked them to send me full details of the events and to include a large scale map of the neighbourhood. I explained that everything is interconnected and therefore the cause of the situation might be miles away. When I received the map, I ascertained through the art of dowsing that there was a violently reversed spiral four and a half miles north west of their house. There was no town or village in that location and I was curious to understand what could be causing the negative vortex. Telephoning them, I asked if I could come to make a tour of the surrounding area. Together we went and searched out the spot that I had found on the map. It was soon apparent what had happened to cause the disharmony.

In the sixteenth and seventeenth centuries, buildings called tithe barns stored the grain that the local farmers paid as a form of tax to the Church. The barns were always built on the point where three of these ley lines intersected, producing a powerful vortex of energy. This had the effect of preserving the grain for long periods of time, which would not have been possible if the barn had been built elsewhere. The barns were built for a specific purpose in the same way that the churches and cathedrals were built for religious purposes, and were also situated on special points on the earth.

In this particular case, a rich businessman from London had purchased a tithe barn, on the exact spot where I had dowsed the problem to be, to use as a country house for parties at weekends. Naturally he had to have a foundation and since the barns always had an earth floor, several inches of concrete had to be poured down. In addition, steel girders were erected where before there was no metal, and water pipes and electrical leads were fed into the rising structure. Worst of all, as a result of the construction, the *flow* of the three lines of energy which were providing a certain life to the cottage and the main house, four and a half miles away, had been blocked. The harmony of the land was reversing itself.

I took fourteen rods and made a pattern around the converted barn. By doing this, I was able to pick up the ley lines from one side of the barn and feed them around to the other side, thus allowing them to flow once again. It did not take long before peace returned to the cottage and the young couple.

In another case an American, his wife and their five children purchased a large farm in the West of England. The man, originally educated at a New England university as an expert in Medieval English, had to learn about farming from scratch and relied mainly on the knowledge of his wife, who had been born and brought up on the land. Between them they did a wonderful job of restoring the farm. They increased the stock of sheep and the prime herd of Jersey cows until it was about eighty-five strong. Suddenly, again for no apparent reason, every new cow that was introduced into the herd developed viral pneumonia. I was called to see if the problem could be solved through the use of geomancy.

Before long I discovered that there was a negative spiral, or vortex, just where the cows waited to go into the milking parlour. I hastened to the farm to see what the cause was, but nothing was apparent on the surface. The cows were waiting to be milked in the usual fashion. It was a warm day in early summer in one of the most beautiful parts of England, but I could sense that something was wrong. With careful dowsing, I found the exact spot where the negative influence existed and asked the farmer and his wife if anything had recently happened near that spot. At first they could not remember anything out of the ordinary, and then the farmer's wife remarked that they had changed the pattern of the milking parlour by concreting the area where the cows were waiting.

The house and farm had both been built in the fifteenth century when concrete was not used. In those days, people used instead, stone, which breathes. As in the last case, the use of the concrete had blocked the lines of energy, resulting in the illness of the Jersey herd. I made a device to free the ley lines and the farm came back into order again. In three weeks, the family went to the market and bought new stock to introduce to the herd. They had no further problems with viral pneumonia.

I thought that I had been able to pass on the basic principles of geomancy to this couple, but obviously, apart from helping the herd, I was being presumptuous. I received another letter. This time, their beautifully matured apple orchard had started to rot and die. They could not determine the reason for this and the advice they had received up to that point had been to no avail. I asked for another map and found the negative spirals. In this case, an underground stream producing negative energy went right through the orchard. Once again I drove down to the West Country.

Walking up the hill from their beautiful farm, I came to a path lying under the downs. At one point I was drawn to a halt just inside the field. Everything felt strange. Returning to the farm, I asked the people to join me to see if they had an explanation for what I felt. It turned out that they had converted an old cottage just near that spot for a new farm manager. In the garden was an original Roman well. The Romans knew a lot about water; each of their wells was dug on the ley lines and were all interconnected. The farmer, in order to save money, or perhaps because he was greedy, had put the sewage pipe into the Roman well instead of making a septic tank which, in England, would have taken much time to get the necessary planning permission and would have cost money.

What had happened? The natural flow of water from the well, which had not been used since the mid-nineteenth century, had been contaminated with sewage. Originally it had been pure water and had fed the apple trees down the hill. In this instance, I was too late. There was nothing that I could do. Sadly all the trees died. Years later, though, I went back and found that the man had finally put in a proper septic tank, in the right place, and had planted a new orchard which was doing well.

One weekend I conducted a workshop on geomancy for thirty-five people in Los Angeles. On the Sunday I took them all to the park to demonstrate the principles that I had been teaching. I stressed how important it was to get permission from the owners of a property before doing geomancy work unless it was a public place, in which case we are all considered to be the custodians of the property. Not realising that it was a holiday, we were surprised to find crowds of people in the park and had to remain 'invisible', as it were, so that we did not attract too much attention. After our picnic, I led the group to a desolate hill where I discovered a negative spiral. On the exact spot of the spiral, we found a dead tree that looked as though it had been struck by lightning. This is not an uncommon sign in geomancy. No one seemed to notice us. I put the rods into the ground to redeem the reversed pattern, we said a prayer together and suddenly a huge flock of birds arrived. Soon we could see children scrambling up through the rough undergrowth towards us. Previously the land had seemed barren and unattractive, unused by both people and animals. As we quietly went down the other side of the hill and looked back, we could hear the happy sounds of voices and singing birds.

I could cite hundreds of such cases as examples of geomancy. The ones that I have chosen, although they may sound different, have something in common running between them. Here is another example.

My family and I had kindly been lent a beautiful house on a mountain above Boulder, Colorado. Beyond the house, but within walking distance, there was a lovely pasture that was part of a national forest. Often the snow, at that height, did not leave until mid-May and so the season for hikers was short. At one time the area had been an extremely prosperous gold mining region. Wherever one walked there were tailings of deserted mines, the entrances to which had been covered with rough boards.

Half way down the pasture, where the view across the Rocky Mountains seemed to stretch out to infinity, was an old burnt out log cabin. The foundations were still there, and the air of violence and sadness was stifling. There were old rusted metal beds lying about, old beer cans, broken glass and rotten mattresses. I resolved to put this to order with the help of the people who were studying with me. Our first priority was to ascertain what had happened there and to discover how far the influence of the fire had spread. I purchased maps of the neighbourhood and, after careful study, found that the effects of the violence had stretched a long way indeed, probably causing trouble on the land up to 32 miles away.

I asked the locals who lived in the mountains what had happened. Mountain people do not talk very much and I had to make my inquiries in such a way that they did not feel suspicious. Eventually I discovered that the cabin had been lived in, about eight years before, by some young people. They had long hair and were part of an overflow of the sixties. There were also some forceful people in that region, called 'red-necks' in America. At that time, the red-necks had tried to get the young people to leave but they refused to go. One night they returned to the cabin and burnt the young people out. As far as I know, nobody was hurt, but the land suffered: as I said before, the land remembers.

One day, with four-wheel trucks, when the snow was still on the ground, we went back to the pasture. We put our rods into the earth at the proper place to correct the flow of energy. We removed all the rubbish from the area and took it to a dump. We added logs for seats, and where before there had been violence, we made a sanctuary out of the chaos. Hikers are attracted to the place now. Perhaps they will never know that someone cared enough to help heal the land.

The events that took place in this case occurred near Sedona in Arizona. A well-known creek ran through the canyon and clusters of charming houses, mainly used by artists, tourists and holiday-makers, lined its banks. Each week the creek was stocked with trout, making the area a popular place for fishermen as well. In every way the land held great charm and there was no obvious reason for disharmony. Yet there was something amiss, particularly in one area. The people who lived there hardly communicated with one another. Even the temperature of the air was colder at that end of the creek, although there was no difference in elevation or in the trees and foliage.

One of the people who lived in that community attended a workshop that I was giving in the town. He informed me of the situation and asked if I would come as a consultant to see if anything could be done to help. As it turned out, it was a perfect opportunity to invite the forty people attending the workshop to the site, for them to see for themselves how a geomancer works. Having already spent one day working with the theories of geomancy, we then got into cars and proceeded to the creek for the fieldwork.

The first thing that I did was to ask the group to be sensitive to all the surroundings, working particularly with their inner senses. I invited them to use their dowsing equipment, if necessary, to see if they could discover any natural disorders, such as the course of the river having been altered or a place where lightning had struck a tree. Both of these could result in a reversed spiral. There are so many factors that must be taken into consideration in dowsing work.

We crossed the river by a little bridge and visited the house of the man who had invited us. Indeed there was a strange atmosphere that was not present at the other end of the creek. Various ideas were presented to me but none of them seemed directly related to the cause of the trouble. I led the group back across the river and we walked on downstream until I could distinctly sense the change of temperature. I felt that the source of the problem lay on the other side of the creek, beyond the place where the path had ended. It was necessary to cross the water, jumping from rock to rock. I left the older people behind, as it was a tricky crossing, and managed to fall in three times myself on the way over!

I found the inevitable negative spiral under a steep, overhanging rock face. This time it was accompanied with the most terrible atmosphere of grief and violence. Some of the people started to cry when I put in a series of three rods to release the trapped energy. As I did so, I had the distinct feeling that on that exact spot someone had either been raped or murdered or both.

The effect of the operation was instantaneous and was witnessed by everyone present. Even the people on the other side of the river, who were waiting but unable to see what was happening, told us that they had felt a tremendous sense of relief at a certain moment. The most obvious physical change was the air temperature which must have risen nearly ten degrees. From the chill came a warmth that seemed kind and inviting.

I did not tell anyone what I had felt but a sensitive English lady in the group turned round and said in front of everyone, "You know, it was so strange and rather frightening. All I sensed when we came upon this spot was the smell of blood and semen . . ."

Nobody will ever know for sure if someone had been raped, the memory would have remained in the exact spot where the deed took place, as indeed every act of violence is registered on Mother Earth. The good news came later when I received a letter saying that there had been remarkable changes in that area of the creek and that people were far more friendly with each other. The effects of that work remain to this day.

I I

Practical 'Home' Work

No book on the subject of healing would be complete without at least one chapter on hospitality and the guest. We take so much for granted during our lives that it is easy to forget what a privilege it is if we are allowed to have a guest in our house, with whom to share a meal or to whom we can offer a bed for the night. In ancient days, the guest was considered almost more important than anything, and the home was organised to receive a guest at any moment. Before the invention of the telephone, it was not necessarily known if and when a guest would arrive and so, not only was a room already prepared with clean sheets on the bed, flowers on the table and a jug of fresh water waiting, but often an extra place was laid on the dining-room table in case a guest would come in time for the meal.

The real reason that this extra care was taken was not just blind superstition, but rather stemmed from a belief that we can never know, precisely, who our guest will be. The physical form, after all, is only a vehicle and, even if we do know the person who comes, we cannot know exactly what that person will bring. Perhaps it will be a message of the utmost importance to help us understand something that has puzzled us for so long, or maybe the guest will be the representation of the Guide who leads all seekers along the Road of Truth. Elijah, in the Bible, is said to represent this Guide.

In many cultures there can be found reference to this strange man, often wearing green, who appears in a mysterious fashion and just as quickly, disappears again. If we are awake to the moment, we can hear what we need to hear. If we are asleep, he goes away without our having heard, and thus we have failed in our role of host or hostess to the very moment itself. We are here to be hosts to and for the moment, as indeed our house is here to receive the guest.

Out of these old traditions came certain rituals and also an outlook towards manners. I feel these manners, which are still with us to this day, not only bear examining but are also necessary for us to put into practice if we truly want to be of service. If we can reverse space and consider how we would like to be treated when we visit someone else's house, it is easier to understand what the guest might need.

The further along the road we go, the more sensitive we become. It is amazing what vibrations can be left in a room, unwittingly, by the people who stayed there before! Anger, grief, fear, all the negative emotions, can be held almost indefinitely in a room if there is no circulation of air or an honest attitude of respect for whoever might come to visit. The guest is the one who suffers the indignity of what is left in a room that has not been cleaned properly.

A home is a healer too, if we consider it. What a wonderful feeling it is, after having been on a long journey, to arrive at someone's house, or at a good hotel, and there is a room to welcome us with a fire in the grate, clean sheets, fresh soap in the bathroom, towels that smell of the breeze in which they were dried and a hot water bottle in the cold of the winter. So much tension is released when we know that we are loved and cared for, and that we are able to stop and rest for a while. Yet, these simple rules are not taught as they used to be and the football game on television seems to have taken precedence over the guest. Although it is true to say that we can be generous with our space and time in the understanding that the more we give, the less we need for ourselves, in reality, we can own neither space nor time, but we can indeed be custodians of it and hosts to it.

Thought-form is a strange phenomenon. It does not

suddenly appear in the atmosphere and then, just as easily, disappear. Thought-forms remain, gathering similar thought-forms, until they are redeemed. A room filled with remorse will attract remorse in the same way that a room with left-over anger will attract a similar thought-form.

There are methods to keep a room clear of unwanted thoughts so that a pure and true welcome can be felt by the guest. The first step is to put our home into a state of order. If order prevails in a room, it does not attract chaos. This can easily be seen in a kitchen. When there is a fine chef, the kitchen is as clean as the bathroom and everything is in order, ready to prepare the meal for the guests. There is as much attention paid to detail as an artist takes with his paints and brushes. The food has been carefully chosen by shopping consciously and, after it is prepared, it is presented in the proper fashion. If the cook is in a bad mood, the emanation goes into the cooking and even sickness can result. Loving care is the definition of fine order for the guest.

As we learn the art of receiving a guest, so we begin to understand the responsibility of being one ourselves. When we enter someone else's house or room, it is important that we leave our own pain behind, unless of course we have been invited to bring it into the room to be dealt with. That is how the old tradition of stepping over the threshold originated. I always stop before opening the door, for a brief moment, to gather myself into a collected state* and then step *over* the threshold rather than on it.

There is another tradition, which has almost been forgotten, that involves space and time. As we are responsible for our own space, so we are responsible for the correct timing. There are day thoughts and night thoughts and they are not the same. In this understanding, if we set the breakfast table before we go to bed at night, we will not only have more time but we will also be prepared for the morning. It is all a question of visualisation, clear intention and loving

*See page 120

attention to each and every detail. Perhaps Elijah will walk in when we are still in our dressing gowns with the table not yet set and no plans made for the first meal of the day! What then?

In the understanding of order, it is important to remember that each room in the house has its own particular function. The house itself is a unity and each room within, whilst serving its own purpose, is also interconnected with every other room. This is often forgotten. The bathroom is seldom recognised as an essential part of the process of transformation. In the same way, the kitchen is not respected for its true purpose. People walk through it, totally asleep, ignoring the cleanliness and concentration that is vital in the preparation of a good meal for the guest. A bedroom too, should be used for the purpose for which a bedroom is intended, and not for massage, healing or therapy. It is no wonder people have such strange dreams! A bedroom implies there is a bed in it upon which people sleep. It is not a place in which we cook or conduct scientific experiments. The bedroom is as sacred as every other room but it has its own function. The guest room is for the guest and the bedroom is for the host and or the hostess. As we define the spaces in our house with respect, so the quality of the functions in each room will be enhanced. Because the home is a unity, disorder in any room will, consequently, affect the whole.

The home is the extension of ourselves. If we live in a world of false glamour, we will produce it in our home. Whereas if we care about our children and our children's children, glamour will mean little to us. If we live in a world of gentle harmony and order, then we will manifest this in our surroundings. A child will remember the environment in which it was born and brought up. It is a splendid challenge to do our best to remember this.

I used to wonder why my mother dusted the furniture, shelves and walls at the same time every morning. It all seemed so unnecessary then, but now it has become part of our own life at home. Remembering the guest, we wash every wall once a week lightly with rose-water, in the knowledge that physical dust collects psychic dust. Who would want to live in a house full of psychic phenomena rather than the loving kindness of a good host and hostess. Windows are meant to be looked out from and so they too need to be cleaned regularly. Shiny surfaces attract radiation, of which there is plenty these days, and it is wise to pay attention to windows, plastic surfaces, mirrors and anything else that might collect this unwanted dust. A mirror is used for the purpose of seeing our own image. If it is covered with splattered toothpaste, it does not fulfil the function for which it was intended. All of these things sound so simple, yet they are important in the beautiful interconnectedness of life. In service, we are asked not to forget or avoid these principles. If we do, it will be like giving someone a wedding cake with a piece taken out of the middle.

There are some useful tips that can be given on how to purify a room. In some countries juniper logs are burned in the fireplace at the end of the day to clear the atmosphere of any lingering thought-forms. In our home, we use a simpler method that has the same effect by taking a tablespoon of Epsom salts, placing it in a pan kept for this purpose, covering the salts with enough rubbing alcohol (obtainable from any chemist) to wet them, setting light to the mixture and then walking in a clockwise direction around the room. It is a wonderful technique to use for children, when they are ill, or in any situation where the room needs cleaning. We often do this in our home the last thing at night, and have given it the nickname 'putting the house to bed'. A pinch of the herb rue, added to the Epsom salts, is excellent in clearing a room where there has been a lot of grief. There are many of these old traditions and sometimes such tips can be used in healing.

Our bodies are composed of at least 64 per cent water and, in respect of this, we should pay particular attention to this element. The fluid in our body needs to be continuously changing if we are to be fit, and able to be of service in any one moment. In the old days, the jug of water beside the bed would be covered either with muslin or lace so that the water would be protected and the air allowed to enter at the same time. The importance of water was understood. How many grains of dust do we drink every night? In this time of history, pure water is something that we can no longer take for granted and, in our gratefulness to be alive, surely we should see every glass of water we take as being sacred.

It is our obligation as a good host or hostess to see that our guest has good water. Maybe there are considerations such as diet or other special needs that we also need to discover in order to be more of service to our guest. We must not presume anything. I was once invited to Texas to give a seminar and a lecture. When I arrived at the house where I was to stay, I was shown to my room, which had a mattress on the floor. Left alone for a little while, I looked around and felt, without any shadow of a doubt, that in no way could I stay there. I asked for someone to come and speak with me, not wanting to be ill-mannered, and explained that I really had to find a more suitable place to rest during that period. When the issue was finally confronted, I was informed that the mattress had been placed on the floor at *exactly* the spot where the hostess, also a therapist, did high colonic irrigations . . . so much for water!

Our home is the extension of ourselves, not only inside but out of doors as well. We are the custodians of the land on which we live. Can we offer our guest the smell of a fresh rose or the sight of a spring garden? We can always have something in our garden to remind us of the beauty of God's creation in the vegetable kingdom. Even if we live in a city, and we do not have a garden, we can always have plants or window boxes. "Look at what I have created for you!" He says, and we forget. We have the tools of healing in our hearts and therefore in our hands. As healers of the world, let us manifest God's beauty on earth, that we may be ready to receive the real Guest. 'I was a hidden treasure and I loved to be known so I created the world that I might be known.' (Haddith (or saying) of the Prophet Mohammed). In these words lies a great message.

12

Conscious Birth, Sex and Death

I would like to dedicate this chapter to the subject of conscious birth, sex and death. After all, when it comes down to it, what else needs to be said about esoteric healing? These three subjects form a beautiful triad around which we weave what is called 'Life', and if we are here to heal, we are also here to become truly conscious human beings.

Today the subject of natural childbirth is talked of widely which is indeed a healthy sign. After all, nothing could be more natural than the act of giving birth. The idea of conscious birth, however, is not often discussed, possibly because of the very meaning of the word 'conscious'. It is a word that is used so frequently, but, I feel, seldom understood. In the dictionary, 'conscious' is described as being 'conscious or aware of one's own existence or environment', and this implies that there is something in us which can be aware. We each have, though often in a dormant state, that which can act as an observer to any given circumstance, whether in the outside world or the world within.

Imagine all that would be necessary in order to have a conscious birth. Who would be the 'observer'? Would it be the mother or father, the doctor or midwife, or others present at the birth? Could this observer be the Invisible Kingdoms who sing at the birth of every child, or is there still another dimension to this idea?

Before we can understand conscious birth, let us first look at consciousness itself. In all inner schools throughout the ages, great stress has been given to the notion that we are 'sleepwalkers', existing on the stage of life, until we are able to wake up to the 'real world' and thus participate in an

entirely different way of life. Of course, we have to realise
that we are asleep before we can wish to wake up, and then,
as in any type of metamorphosis, the waking process can be
painful.

Just as a mother giving birth to her child experiences a
certain type of pain, so we, in a sense, are born into the 'real
world', and the pain that we feel hides a joy that makes it
easier to bear. In fact, if we could only know it, this is what
conscious suffering is all about in everyday life. We bear the
pain of suffering, physically, emotionally and even spirit-
ually, gladly, knowing it is a part of the growth process as
we emerge from the darkness of the cave into true light.
Jesus once said in *The Apocryphal Acts of John,* 'Ye thought
that I suffered, but I suffered not . . .'

True healing is very much to do with becoming conscious. A real healer is able to add the necessary ingredient to
a human being's life so that he or she is finally able to wake
up to what is occurring in the present moment, without
being biased by what has happened in the past. A person
who is awake is free, whereas a person who is asleep is still
tied to the continuously turning wheel of suffering.

'Polish the mirror of your heart' is a great Sufi saying, but
it is difficult to polish a heart that is full of remorse, anger
and bitterness. Such a heart needs to be 'free' and then it is
up to us to keep it polished so that it can reflect the needs of
the moment. Practices such as conscious breathing, concentration on light and visualisation of beauty can help clear
the patterns of the past as well as providing a suitable polish,
but it is our responsibility to do the work. No one else can
do it for us.

The observer is part of ourselves, as so many dormant
aspects are, all of which need to be awakened in order that
we become complete human beings. The observer becomes
real in us as our intention to live becomes clearer and clear.
Eventually it is possible to say, 'I am that which observes
and that which is observed.'

To build in this observer, the first effort we need to make
is to ask ourselves, in all sincerity, whether we actually have
a real question. I do not mean the normal, run-of-the-mill
questions that we ask each day, but something much deeper
and more profound. We could, for example, ask ourselves,
every waking moment, 'What is the purpose of life on
earth?' or 'What is our individual purpose of life on earth?'
or even 'Do we have a purpose?' We have all asked such
questions but they are usually born out of despair, when
something has happened to us which is unpleasant, or sad,
or at times of great grief or mourning.

To be able to ask questions such as these, we must be clear
of all that veils us. The fog that haunts us must go through a
polished heart, for only then can we ask a question about
conscious birth, sex and death, and, at the same time, be
open and able to receive an answer.

The question is vitally important. If we live in the question, we are in the river that leads back to the ocean, whence
we came. It is the fastest part of the river and yet also the
calmest. The purpose of a healer (and are we not all healers?), is to leave us with a question and not an answer. In the
same way that no two experiences are alike, no one but
ourself can find the answer for us. The answer will then be
our own and part of our living reality. The Divine Guidance, it is said, is to lead us to the point of perplexity.

When we realise that we do not have a real question, we
can then begin to find one. Initially this seems easy, but the
more we work with the nature of the question and the
deeper we go, the more we understand that it is also a matter
of where we ask the question from. If our question comes
from intellectual reasoning, we will either get an intellectual
answer, a headache, or no answer at all. If we ask from our
limited ego consciousness, then we will only increase the
power of our ego and are apt to get psychically as fat as a
balloon. It is only when our whole being resounds to the
question which comes from the heart itself, that, as time

unfolds and we become more and more conscious, we can become the instruments in a symphony. Then, as Mevlana Jelaluddin Rumi, the great Sufi poet and mystic of the thirteenth century once said, 'We are the flutes, but the music is Thine'.

As we live in the question each moment, our own question, we start to develop true will. Ralph Waldo Emerson said about will: 'It is the sustaining, coercive and ministerial power – the police officer in man'. Without will, we are bound hand and foot in the chains of fate, and are seldom able to embrace the arms of Destiny, who waits for us always with loving care. With will, we can be conscious at last.

Conscious birth is part of the cycle of life which starts with the point of conception, and here we are talking about a couple who are conscious at the point of conception. Often women know when they have conceived. Sometimes men are also awake to that moment although the experience is more rare, I believe. When my second son was conceived, I can remember a brilliant light filling the whole room. It is in the degree of passion at the moment of conception that a pattern is fixed for the embryo of the child. For, unlike an animal, a human being has both instinct and consciousness.

Let us now look at the ideal conditions for conscious birth. During the months of pregnancy, a new rate of vibration is felt in the family and deep respect is paid to it. The woman, after the fifth month, spends a special part of each day quietly listening to her favourite music, looking at beautiful pictures and savouring the delights around her – the flowers in the garden, the butterflies, the birds and all of the beautiful world that God has given us. The woman and her friends do everything they can to see that she has no cause for worry. She has done her pre-natal experiences, a room has been set aside for the child-to-come and everything is made ready. The walls are washed with rose-water, the space is made to be as receptive as is humanly possible, and finally the labour commences.

The man, by this time, has gained will, through his sacrifice to the question, and is therefore conscious of the present moment. Both of them have studied conscious breathing and the rhythm of the Mother's breath*. He stands at her right side, during the birth, erect and with absolute confidence. How a woman respects this!

They are not just concentrating on the birth of the baby, but are also present for the emergence of a *being,* whose presence will be seen in the form of this little child. Great emphasis is given to the meaning of the 'agreement' to this being who is emerging into this world from a much higher world. It will be a stranger in a strange land and will need to be recognised for what it is, to be welcomed into a world of trials and tribulations, a world that is absolutely necessary for its own completion. It is difficult not to be sentimental when a beautiful little child is suddenly with us and easy to forget that what we see is only the vehicle for what we cannot see. Sentimentality is the greatest enemy of love.

The play continues . . . the labour increases, the midwife or doctor is there to give assistance and everyone works as a team in this great event. Imagine what we would all have felt like if our parents were as present in the moment as I am suggesting we need to be as healers of the world.

The moment arrives, the baby is born and it is laid on the mother's stomach to get used to this new rhythm of breath, this new air. Already it is used to the Mother's Breath, but now it is in a world where not everyone knows of this breath, and it is aware of this. It has landed on the planet, and because of all the conscious preparation, it knows that it is loved, and that it is welcomed unconditionally.

There is quietness in the room. Everyone present has been instructed in the breathing process and in how to visualise light energy for the child. Little by little the umbilical cord starts to go milky white, and, after a certain time, even up to forty minutes, when it is sensed by the father and the

*See page 109

midwife that all is ready, the father cuts the cord himself, in full consciousness, accepting his responsibility, and offering the child into the lap of the Divine. Consciousness – the awareness of all that is both in the room and in the world around – pervades the moment. It is the beginning.

Just as conscious birth is a cosmic event in which everyone shares, seen most clearly in the birth of Christ, so is the act of making love. Yet how seldom do we ever hear it said that the act of sex, of making love, that is, making love possible on earth, is the most sacred act there is in our relative world. The act of sex is not just for the release of tension, nor indeed solely for the procreation of the species. It is far bigger and wider than that. It is a cosmic play, a carnival which brings in all of the invisible worlds, if we could only know and recognise them. It is a ballet, an opera; it is a symphony and a passionate acceptance of life itself.

Only through endless preparation and practice are the three great mysteries of birth, sex and death unfolded to us. Therein lies an enormous question: are we ready for sex? Although it is not difficult to see how much study it takes to become a master carpenter or doctor, a musician or painter, a composer or a conductor, we still often presume the act of making love, and thus it may not always be conscious. It may produce a high degree of sensitivity and loving attention, but if it is truly conscious, then it is an act that blends all the worlds together, the worlds of thought and feeling, the worlds of aspiration and motivation, the kingdoms of the mineral world, the vegetable world, the animal world and mankind. It is a vast and wonderful story.

In the same way that no two people are alike and no two thumbprints are alike, all over the world, so no two experiences can be alike. What, therefore, can be written about conscious sex? Are we not consecrating that which is not yet formed, rather like consecrating unleavened bread? Perhaps this is a strange analogy, but that is exactly what it is all about. For every conscious act of sex, whether or not the

wife conceives at that time, a child is born in love somewhere in the world.

Conscious sex produces objective hope, that is, not hope
from ignorance, but true hope from knowledge itself. Two
human beings who realise the true significance of conscious
sex are the central characters in the play called 'life'. We all
turn to those in love, to those who have totally committed
themselves to each other and to a life of service. There is a
radiance about them, something that shines forth like a
beacon to those shipwrecked on the cliffs of opportunity.

It can be said that commitment produces hazard and yet,
without hazard there is no true love. Commitment shows
us what we need to understand and then it is up to us
whether we face the trials that are really necessary for the
transformation process to take place. Indeed, it can be truly
said that without true commitment there is merely the
turning around, the bubbling and ferment of history repeating itself. Conscious sex produces brotherhood, a true
brotherhood which nothing can destroy for it is real. It faces
life as it faces death, treating, as Rudyard Kipling once said,
those 'two imposters just the same'.

Agreement is a stronger word than God. It is through the
agreement of two conscious human beings that conscious sex
is made possible, not just for this time but for the generations
to come. Agreement can produce further and further degrees
of agreement until two souls in two bodies become one soul
in two bodies, one soul in eternal love. That is what conscious sex is all about. It is nothing less than this.

How do we set about knowing how to have conscious
sex, or to make love consciously? There is no difference in
either birth, sex or death. It is a question of understanding,
of sacrifice, of a deep inner love and conviction that we are
indeed here for a purpose with every nerve and sinew, every
breath and movement and every intention and agreement
that we can muster within, through our practices and training, taken from the Highest Source that we can envisage.

Let us look once again at this great triad of birth, sex and death. Which comes first? It is said that the cause is the effect of its own effect and perhaps herein lies the answer. There is the eternal recurrence of life, this miracle spiralling its way towards completion. No one can say where it starts or where it will end since there really is neither beginning nor end. There is only the appearance of an interruption in cycles. I fear we are frightened of death, and yet, in fear there can be no knowledge. In knowledge there is no death. There is the pure energy of consciousness, carrying with it higher and higher degrees of energy from worlds beyond any possible imagination we can have until we are awake, free and able to understand.

Healing is to do with understanding in Truth, for love and knowledge are the two arms of the heart. The understanding of the purpose of being conscious at the three great moments of this life's cycle can never be underestimated. Hell is when we are not in the present moment. It is not some strange kingdom in a world after death. The Hereafter is *here* after we have finally woken to eternity in the present moment.

A short time ago we were invited to be with a young friend who was dying from an incurable disease. He was in intensive care and on life-support systems. By the time we reached the hospital, he was very close to death. I said to him, "My friend, there are only two things I wish to say to you. First of all, do you know that you are loved?" This is surely the first step towards true healing and is often forgotten. "Yes", he replied, and I knew that his answer was genuine. "Now", I said, "after all these years of training with the breath and learning how to be conscious, will you please be conscious on your last breath and remember the *sound* of the words in *The Invisible Way,*★ 'I love you – there is nothing else.' If you can do this, then your memory will go on forever." We bade him farewell, and as we were
★See *The Invisible Way*, Element Books

going out of the door, I turned back for a moment and, pointing upwards said, "See you up there!" It was a very moving experience for I was both laughing and crying at the same time. He smiled with great dignity and managed to say, "Be careful, I might be back sooner than you think. If you both decide to have a child, I might just pop in!"

In that little saga lies a real thread of truth. Our friend died consciously and in that valiant effort, somewhere a child was conceived in love and would be born consciously. Can we see the immensity of this understanding? Any single conscious act of birth, sex or death immediately produces in someone else the possibility of reaching a higher level of being. It is through the sacrifice of those who have gone before, that we exist at all, and it is through those who have become awake in this lifetime that we have the chance to become awake ourselves.

The question arises once more as to how we build in this observer, or how do we awaken what is already there. Again I would stress that practices are essential. They become our part of the bargain of life. We are given it to live. The paradox is that we cannot die to the illusion of our separateness from the Unity until we are awake, and we cannot be truly awake until we die to the illusion itself! Indeed, all life is a paradox, a play, a masquerade, and it is what we make of it that truly counts. If we die consciously, then someone else is liable to repeat that same performance, for in Reality there is only One Absolute Being, and we are just parts of the Whole, manifestations of the Divine Unity.

Herein lies another paradox. Since in reality there is no death, how then can we be conscious at the moment of transition? The answer is to do with the breath. How many of us have ever been taught how to breathe? We come into life on the breath and we go out of life on the breath, but so often we presume what we are given. We presume the seasons, we presume our own gender, we presume other people's genders, and their families, and their lives.

We presume, not realising that no two people can think alike and therefore it is so important that respect comes first in our relationships. Respect comes before love. Love is pure energy, manifested in this world to help continue what the late G.I. Gurdjieff called 'The Experiment of Life on Earth'.

It is through the realisation of breath, rather than the presumption that it will go on forever, that we come to this great mystery of something that is called death. To me, death is not a mystery. It is a miracle, a wonderful and beautiful miracle whereby people are taken out of a world of trial and suffering and yet, at the same time, are here with us always. Did not Jesus say, "I will be with you always, even unto the end of time."

I have no fear of death. The death process may be somewhat painful and difficult, but that too is a challenge. Some of the greatest masters have consciously chosen to put themselves through enormous suffering, not for themselves, but in order to redeem others of unnecessary suffering in their own lives. There are many examples. The agony of death in true consciousness is the implantation of mystery and glorification in the worlds to come. This is a challenge that we can meet. We are here to heal, and these sacred acts of birth, sex and death are the keys to true freedom.

13

The Practice Programme

INTRODUCTION

It takes practice to gain mastery over any skill, whether it be carpentry, architecture, medicine, music, design or any other field of excellence, and through that skill, we then have a frame in which we can serve other people. We are all here to heal, as conscious beings, but in order to become conscious, we have to give our part in the bargain of life. Understanding comes through practice and patience. As I have already stated, it is only through endless preparation and practice, that the three great mysteries of life, conscious birth, sex and death, are unfolded to us. We cannot just presume that we know. Dedicated practice develops will and with will we are able to offer our lives to a life of service.

The purpose of the practice programme is to enable us to be balanced on the physical and the subtle levels of our being so that we can be 'here' to heal. True healing can only occur in the present moment. These practices help us not to identify with but rather to consciously participate in life. The exercises are not to get us 'high'. Through conscientious attention to them, however, they can help us to build a more solid foundation upon which we can serve the planet and our fellow human beings.

This twenty-four day programme is designed to help keep the life force flowing regularly. Correct attitude is all-important. So often people do certain practices in order to escape from an emotional or mental situation, but if they are used in this manner, they can have the opposite effect. The best way of approaching such a programme is to look at it as one would look at preventive medicine. If our teeth are not cleaned regularly, then we may develop cavities and gum disease, whereas if we keep up a regular programme of cleaning, we save ourselves a lot of trouble and money.

This particular programme can be done in conjunction with any other exercises or practices that people may be involved with. After the cycle has been completed, any or all of the practices can be continued. The reason for the length of time that I have advocated is to do with the time it takes to help clear the toxins that are so easily collected in the various levels of our being.

It is important to set aside at least twenty minutes a day, while participating in the programme, for good physical exercise, whether it be jogging, walking, playing tennis or some other favourite activity. The type of exercise is not as important as the right intention lying behind it. We try to be conscious with each and every breath. If it were walking we had chosen for the day, then we would try to extend ourselves as much as possible without unnecessary strain, attempting to be aware with every step we take. We wish to be in balance on all levels and to be so attuned that we can know what we are doing, at any one moment, and in any given situation, as well as realising the implications of any action that we make. Without conscious exercise, it is difficult to maintain this balance.

It can be helpful to make an agreement to participate in the programme with others since agreement in action is half the battle won. Real agreement produces a certain type of energy. If one's friend or partner follows the same programme and time schedule, it can be beneficial to both, even though the practices are geared essentially to the individual. There are no group practices mentioned in this particular programme. However, each individual is unique within Unity, and therefore, practices can be done with others who have been drawn together with the same purpose in heart and mind, even though the individual practice may be different as, for example, in the decision-making exercise.

It is best that personal experiences are not discussed

with anyone. There is always the danger that someone, not having had what they consider to be a valid 'experience' might try to copy the experience of another and then it would not be real. No two people can ever have the same experience in anything. There may be similarities, but that is all. We are all unique, with no two thumb-prints alike, so how then can we have the same experience as another!

Finally, although this cannot be forced, I firmly advocate that if for some reason more than two days in a row are missed during the twenty-four day cycle, the course is started over again from the beginning. I remember being told in one of the schools with which I studied, that if any of us ever missed more than two weekly classes in a row, we would be sent away to consider what the *real* reason for our absence was, rather than the apparent reason. One young man had broken his leg in a skiing accident and his excuse was hospitalisation. "Ah", said our teacher, "but *why* did you break your leg? You haven't broken it before, that I know of. Because there is no such thing as chance, it must have been that your intention to attend the classes was not strong and clear enough. You were merely finding a good way to try to wriggle out of the results of a weak intention." In this case, the man understood, was allowed back and everything settled down.

Let us remember once more that great Sufi saying, 'Keep your intention before you at every step you take. You wish for freedom and you must never forget it.'

BREATHING PRACTICE OR THE MOTHER'S BREATH

Method

Sit in a hard-backed chair, feet flat on the floor, with heels together and toes apart forming a triangle. Legs should be uncrossed. Arms should be relaxed and if possible in an unstressed position; hands should rest on knees. The solar plexus has two subsidiary centres which are located in the knees. The knees are highly sensitive instruments. If you focus your attention on your knees while blindfolded, you can sense that the knees send out a beam of energy. You will not walk into the wall due to the inner sense that comes from the area of your knees.

Keeping your back straight, without forcing it, will allow the flow of energy to move as it should. With practice your back will straighten naturally. Do this exercise for about ten minutes and no longer. It can be done several times a day with safety.

Before you start the conscious breathing exercise, visualise the most beautiful object in nature you can imagine. It could be a plant, a tree, a waterfall, the sea, or whatever means something real to you. All of these practices are to help us to see God's beauty and to help us live beautiful lives.

For this practice, the eyes can be open or closed. Either way, focus on a point approximately eight feet in front of you. If your eyes are closed then put the picture of whatever you've chosen eight feet in front of you through visualisation. If you are focusing on an object, put it as close to eight feet away from you as you can. *Do not meditate on a candle in this practice.* This is very important. The object of the visualisation is to help you focus your attention, not to meditate on the object itself.

Now we come to this sacred rhythm, this 7 – 1 – 7 – 1 – 7 rhythm, about which I have spoken in former books and which I have been teaching for so long. The rhythm came from ancient Egypt and there are many hieroglyphics showing how this practice, and others, are done. The method is simple though initially it may seem difficult since we are used to just breathing without any form of attention or consciousness. You may notice that the rhythm corresponds exactly to the octave in music.

First, find a point in the centre of your solar plexus area, and also a point in the centre of the chest, which we call the Heart Centre. You are going to breathe into the solar plexus, and then radiate out breath from the heart.

Please remember in working with the 7 – 1 – 7 – 1 – 7 that it is not the speed that counts, be it slow or relatively fast. It is the actual number of counts that we are talking about. Choose the speed that suits you. Breathe into the solar plexus. As you breathe, bring in all the elements of the earth, the minerals (you can even breathe in vitamins by choice if you wish!) and fill yourself with all that the body and its subtle counterparts need. Do not be embarrassed about taking what you need in the understanding that all this is done in the name of service.

Having breathed in for the count of seven, pause for one count and at the same time, bring your attention to the centre of the chest. Then breathe out for the count of seven. As you breathe out, radiate love and goodwill to all mankind from the centre of the chest, as if you are a lighthouse for the ships that are entering the harbour. Be sure to radiate not just in front of you, but also behind, and in all the six directions. At this point, there is a tremendous sense of wonder and gratitude in the realisation that, indeed, we are able to serve our fellow human beings and the planet itself.

We can choose the quality of the air that we breathe. As you progress in the practice, through correct visualisation, you can breathe the air that is circulating in certain sacred areas of the planet. You can breathe the air in Jerusalem, or Glastonbury, without leaving the chair upon which you are sitting.

The last step in the exercise, which, after all, is an alchemical process, is the refining of the breath. Begin taking only as much breath as you actually need and are given. This should require as little effort as the fluttering of a butterfly's wings. There is no more need to force the breath. In a sense, at this stage, you are not breathing. Rather, you are being breathed. Breath is Life! This is the still point in a waiting world.

To complete the practice, return to the senses. As in other practices, feel your body and take responsibility for it once more. Be awake to the room or the surroundings and finally agree that you have fulfilled what you set out to do.

THE END OF DAY CLEARING EXERCISE

It is inevitable that throughout our day there is a build-up of unredeemed thought-forms which can be carried over into the next day. It is important that we clear these thoughts so they do not become our motivators. This twenty-four day programme is geared to both bringing us into the present moment and increasing the flow of life force. In this context, many people have said that the clearing exercise has been one of the most valuable for them.

Method

Directly before going to sleep, lie on your back in a relaxed manner, arms by your side and legs uncrossed. Breathe deeply and rhythmically. Now, placing your attention on the soles of your feet, consciously remember the moment that you got out of bed in the morning. Try to visualise your impressions at that time. The key word in this practice is gratefulness. Our task is to try consciously to have a sense of gratitude for every memory as it arises.

Slowly bringing your attention up the legs and through the body, remember as much as you can of what happened during the day. Your feet will represent the first moment that you got out of bed since they were the first part of your body to touch the floor. Do not judge whatever memories arise. There might be so-called unpleasant experiences but since life itself is the only real teacher, it is experience that counts. There is always something that can be learned from our experiences.

When you have brought your attention through the body and have remembered all that you can, repeat the practice two more times. This is to be quite sure that what is left within is a sense of gratitude, rather than one of bitterness, envy, pride or any of the other negative emotions that beset us so often. This may take a little practice but in a few days, you will see how the clearing practice helps your next day in the right manner.

When everything has been completed, make a decision as to the exact time you will get up the next day and then have a restful night.

REJUVENATION EXERCISE

Many of us have 'low' periods in the day when it is difficult to get things done. Particularly if we live in a city where the air is so badly polluted and there is noise and traffic to contend with, it is useful to have tools to help us. This practice is one such tool.

Method

Take a bowl of water, or the sink if it is big enough, and fill it with cold water. The depth is important. When placing your hand flat into the bottom of the bowl, the water should reach up exactly to the centre of the wrist bone.

Place a copper penny at the bottom of the bowl between the two hands with the thumbs and index fingers touching to form a triangle. The bowl should be at such a height that when bending over, the back can be kept as straight as possible from the waist up.

Breathe in to the count of seven as you slowly bend over the bowl, pause for one count, and then breathe out for seven counts as you return to a standing position once again. Do this seven times and then reverse the breathing pattern so that you breathe out as you bend over, and you breathe in as you come back to the standing position.

BREATHING PRACTICE — STANDING POSITION

The purpose of this practice is to increase the flow of life-force as well as improve your power of concentration. It can also help to open the blocked channels in the etheric, or subtle bodies.

For this practice, you will need a thick piece of white card about a foot square, in the middle of which you have drawn a black disc about the size of a penny. The disc needs to be sharply defined so it is best to use ink or paint. The card is placed at eye level on a wall about six feet in front of where you are standing.

Before commencing, do a few stretches to get the body moving and then take up your position six feet in front of the disc. The arms should be by your sides, the body in an alert but relaxed position with the back straight. The legs should be slightly apart. If you find that there is more energy passing through the right nostril, then the right foot should be slightly forward. If there is more energy in the left nostril, then it is the left foot that should be slightly ahead of the other. If the breath is perfectly balanced, then the legs should be parallel with the feet slightly apart. In your hands you are holding a portion of broom handle, approximately eight inches long, one piece in each hand. The entire practice consists of only twelve breath cycles.

Method

Facing the disc on the white card and remembering the breathing rhythm of 7 – 1 – 7 – 1 – 7, breathe into the solar plexus on the count of seven. At the same time, slowly rise up on the balls of your feet and clench the wood in your hands. The rest of your body, if possible even the arms above the elbow, should be quite relaxed. After the seven counts, slowly start to relax your hands and wrists and return to the original position. At the same time, breathe out light in all directions from the centre of your chest area.

As instructed, this practice should only be done for twelve breath cycles and preferably should be done before meals. When the practice has been completed, wrap the pieces of wood carefully in a cloth, and put them in a safe place. Over a period of time, they will gain a great deal of magnetic energy and so should not be treated lightly. To complete the exercise, do a few more stretches and then continue with whatever you were doing.

DECISION PRACTICE

Most of us are never taught that there are two types of thought pattern. There are night thoughts as well as day thoughts, just as there are daydreams and the dreams we have at night. This is important to understand. There are obviously things that we do after the sun goes down which are better attended to at that time rather than during the day. It is the same the other way round.

Through this practice, little by little, we begin to build a blend of these two patterns of thought. This has the effect of providing us with a certain type of will which we did not have before. The simplicity of the practice should not mislead us into trying to make it more complicated than advocated, for the sake of getting something extra out of it. All of these practices are essentially simple. I learned a version of this one when I was in the boy scouts!

Method

Before retiring to bed, having put yourself into a calm frame of mind with the use of the breathing practice, visualise something that needs to be completed in your house or garden that will take no longer than five minutes. The task should be extremely simple, such as cleaning a pair of shoes, or emptying out a cupboard that you have been avoiding for so long. In the garden, you might weed a border, trim a hedge, or simply sweep the pavement. There is nothing new in what you will be doing since these things are done every day. However, the key words here are decision and visualisation and they are used to bring us into a greater state of awareness.

The next step in the exercise is to visualise, *in detail,* the job that you decided to do the next day. You need to be meticulous about this visualisation. For example, if your decision was to clean a pair of shoes, then you would visualise where the shoes were, see yourself getting them out of the wardrobe and placing them in a suitable spot. You would then see yourself putting down a newspaper, and taking out the polish and brushes from where they were kept. Proceed with the visualisation until the cleaning process saw its completion, finally returning the shoes to the wardrobe, the polish and brushes to their cupboard and throwing away the newspaper.

A portion of us will try to resist this decision that we have made, providing all sorts of excuses as to why this seems so trite, or by saying that there is no time. This is exactly the part of us that needs to come under the command of the Higher Self until it is willing to co-operate in every way. At the end of this visualisation, therefore, try to be sure that all of you is willing to complete the task the next day.

The second part of the practice is done in the morning and is, of course, completing the visualisation that was done the night before. First you re-make the decision to do the task and then remember all the steps in the process and the time that it is to be done. At that time, follow all the details that you visualised until you have finished the job. When the task is over, agree that you have completed it and the time and in the manner that you decided and then go about your business.

Again I stress that the task should take no longer than five minutes. Every act should be an act of awareness as you observe the body fulfilling the job that was started in the mind, employing the pattern of night thoughts.

PEBBLE IN THE WATER EXERCISE

However simple this practice may appear to be, do not underestimate it. The object is to bring about a very deep understanding of the nature of vibration and emanation. People so often say that someone has 'good vibes'. They do not realise that what they are talking about are people's *emanations*. Emanations come out of the rate of someone's vibrations and not the other way around.

Drop a pebble in a clear pool of water. The rings that you see on the surface are dependent on the size of the pebble and the height from which it is dropped. Believe it or not, the rings that appear are also dependent on the *mood,* and the state of the person who drops the pebble. Try it!

The reason for this practice is to prove that *you* are, as it were, the water, the pebble and the person tossing it. After all, it is a scientific fact that we are at least made up of 64 per cent water. As we discover which part of us is the pebble, so we can understand the nature of these emanations.

Method

Sit very still and follow the breath with the usual 7 – 1 – 7 – 1 – 7 rhythm. Close your eyes slowly and carefully, withdrawing your senses from the outer world. Imagine that you are sitting by the side of a perfectly still lake. There is no wind to ruffle the surface of the water and everything is completely still and quiet. It is early morning. Choose a smooth, round pebble from the side of the lake. Feel it in your hands. Polish it with your fingers and your palms. Weigh it, know every portion of it. Become very fond of it.

The next thing you will be asked to do is to throw your pebble into the lake in such a way as to cause the least possible commotion. There should be scarcely the sound of a splash. Get yourself ready, poised and balanced. When the time is right, throw the pebble at the angle you choose, watch its flight as it arcs up and then down into the lake. Now sit quietly and follow the rings that emanate out from the centre until the lake is quite still again. You will see how they get wider and wider, yet the memory remains at the point where the pebble touched the water. The memory remains because you choose it to; otherwise it would be forgotten forever.

When the lake has become perfectly still, observe your breathing once again. Feel your body in a collected state where you are sitting, and then, carefully open your eyes and observe your surroundings. Note if they seem different from what they were.

Once this practice is understood, it is amazing what effect you can have in a chaotic restaurant, supermarket or bank!

THE MIRROR EXERCISE

It is often said that 'Everything is done with mirrors'. What we apparently see in this relative world is, of course, a mere reflection of the world of becoming. This, in turn, is a reflection of a yet higher world, and the process goes on *ad infinitum*. When we begin to understand, we find that this passing world, in which we stay for a little while, is only part of the great process of life. Just as there is life on earth, which is mainly organic, so there is a higher life, a higher state of evolution that we call 'Conscious Evolution'. This is not understood by many since most of the time we live only in the world that we observe around us and that we imagine to be *real*. In reality this world is a reflection.

We can look at it this way. What would be the point of the Sun if there was no Earth upon which to shine its light? In our solar system the sun is created to give light to this earth, and everything being interconnected, the reflection upon the earth returns to the Source of all Light. In the same way, the Inner Work is sometimes called, 'The Path of Return'.

Now the sun takes its light from another sun, in another galactic system, and it in turn takes its light from yet a further sun, each light being more and more refined. The light behind the sun cannot be seen with the naked eye, but it can be felt and sensed with the heart. It is sometimes called 'Black Light' since we cannot see black with our normal eyes. Keeping this in mind, the mirror exercise is like the story of *Alice Through the Looking Glass*.

Method

Visualise seven mirrors in front of you, just as if they were propped on a table with you in front of them.

1 Look at yourself in the first mirror just as you appear to be. See what you look like.

2 Look at the seventh mirror. I suspect you'll find nothing there.

3 Look at yourself in the first mirror.

4 Look at the second mirror – at every physical problem you may have. See them in the second mirror, having accepted the first mirror.

5 Now turn the first mirror around to face the second mirror. (Physical pain facing what you thought you were).

6 Look into the third mirror. This will be your sexual life, completely honestly, faithfully and of course not just the physical act. Let it face the mirror before.

7 Now turn the first mirror back to face yourself and see if you look any different.

8 Now take the second mirror facing the first mirror as before and turn the third mirror to face the fourth mirror. Our prayer is to be purified.

9 Look at your emotional being in the fourth mirror... the beginning of the higher emotions being activated by the mirror before.

10 Take the first four mirrors and face yourself. We are going to go through them. Having faith in your Lord, go through the first four mirrors. Go through time and space, already free of the lower emotions, and distil an aspect of yourself.

11 Take the fifth and the sixth mirrors together, still facing yourself, letting go of all concepts of yourself. If you are in trouble, see the first mirror at the beginning again.

12 Turn around the fifth mirror to face the sixth mirror

and then the sixth to face the seventh. Turn around the seventh mirror to face the endless possibility.

13 Let the Light behind the Sun illuminate the seventh mirror.

14 Turn the seventh mirror to the sixth, illuminating it with the Light behind the Sun and through the sixth into the fifth mirror.

15 Then turn all the mirrors at once, that you may look through the seven mirrors or seven veils of life.

16 Feel your body just as it is before opening your eyes or completing the contemplation.

THE PRESENT MOMENT EXERCISE

Obviously without being in the present moment we will not do very well as healers. Either we will be working from opinions based on the past, or day-dreaming into the future. Thus any practices which help us to come into the present moment with every part of our being, and with every cell of our bodies, will be beneficial, not to ourselves alone, but for the good of the whole. It is almost our obligation to 'collect' ourselves and thus be able to serve better.

The mind is like a wild horse which has to be tamed and made our friend. Time can then be on our side. As we all no doubt know, it is the mind, with all its many and compli-cated facets, plus the emotions, which constitute most of our physical illness. We also know that every cell of the body has consciousness and is continuously being changed. In order for there to be proper flow within us, the mind has to be harnessed and the body and its organs reminded of their proper function. This exercise is geared to this end.

The present moment exercise can be practised at any time that you feel it is necessary. After completing the twenty-four day programme, it should be possible to be in the present moment with just the use of breath, the visualisation of the practice and the memory of the work you have done with it.

Before any healing work is done, whether to do with human beings, animals, birds, the vegetable kingdom or the planet itself, become aware of your surroundings and what is going on around you. Now put your attention on the top of the head. Very carefully, relax all the muscles in the head from the top downwards, paying particular attention to the temples, the eyes and eyelids, the cheeks and jaw and even the tongue. Do not miss anything! When you have done this, then bring this energy of attention down the right side of your body from the neck and the shoulders. Start with the tension in the shoulders and shoulder blades, letting go of any tension that you find there. Bring your attention down the right arm, remembering the elbows, the wrists, the hand as a whole and each finger individually. Now return to the right shoulder and bring this attention down the right side of the body, again noting if there is any tension. You can also add the dimension of light to the organs and other parts of the inside of the body. Move on down the right side through the right buttock, the hip, the thigh, not forgetting the knee, and then down through the leg, to the ankle, the foot and the toes. When this is completed, return to the left shoulder and repeat the practice, moving down the left arm first and then down the left side. Finally bring your attention once more to the top of the head and, as though with one sweep, bring light and relaxation to the whole of the body.

If your eyes have been closed, open them very slowly and look around once again at the space in which you are sitting. Sense how you are feeling; watch the rise and fall of your breath and be very still. There is nothing to fear; there is only to BE.

SUNDAY	Day 1 MONDAY	Day 2 TUESDAY
Prepare	Decision (5)	Decision (5)
BREAKFAST	BREAKFAST	BREAKFAST
	Present Moment (8)	Breathing (1) Present Moment (8)
LUNCH	LUNCH	LUNCH
		Breathing (1)
DINNER	DINNER	DINNER
Decision to commence	Decision (5) Clearing (2)	Decision (5) Clearing (2)

Key to numbers:
(1) Breathing practice
(2) Clearing exercise
(3) Rejuvenation exercise (whenever needed)
(4) Breathing practice (standing)
(5) Decision exercise
(6) Pebble in the water exercise
(7) Mirror exercise
(8) Present Moment exercise

Day 3 WEDNESDAY	Day 4 THURSDAY	Day 5 FRIDAY	Day 6 SATURDAY
Decision (5)	Decision (5) Standing Breathing (4)	Decision (5)	Decision (5)
BREAKFAST	BREAKFAST	BREAKFAST	BREAKFAST
Breathing (1) Present Moment (8) Standing Breathing (4)	Breathing (1) Present Moment (8)	Breathing (1) Present Moment (8)	Breathing (1) Present Moment (8)
LUNCH	LUNCH	LUNCH	LUNCH
Breathing (1) Standing Breathing (4)	Standing Breathing (4)	Breathing (1)	
DINNER	DINNER	DINNER	DINNER
Decision (5) Clearing (2)	Decision (5) Clearing (2)	Pebble (6) Decision (5) Clearing (2)	Decision (5) Clearing (2)

Day 7 SUNDAY	Day 8 MONDAY	Day 9 TUESDAY
Decision (5) Standing Breathing (4)	Decision (5) Mirror (7)	Decision (5)
BREAKFAST	BREAKFAST	BREAKFAST
Breathing (1) Present Moment (8) Standing Breathing (4)	Breathing (1) Present Moment (8)	Breathing (1) Present Moment (8)
LUNCH	LUNCH	LUNCH
Standing Breathing (4)	Breathing (1)	Breathing (1)
DINNER	DINNER	DINNER
Decision (5) Clearing (2)	Decision (5) Clearing (2)	Decision (5) Clearing (2)

Key to numbers:
(1) Breathing practice
(2) Clearing exercise
(3) Rejuvenation exercise (whenever needed)
(4) Breathing practice (standing)
(5) Decision exercise
(6) Pebble in the water exercise
(7) Mirror exercise
(8) Present Moment exercise

Day 10 WEDNESDAY	Day 11 THURSDAY	Day 12 FRIDAY	Day 13 SATURDAY
Decision (5) Standing Breathing (4)	Decision (5)	Decision (5)	Decision (5)
BREAKFAST	BREAKFAST	BREAKFAST	BREAKFAST
Breathing (1) Present Moment (8) Standing Breathing (4)	Breathing (1) Present Moment (8)	Breathing (1) Present Moment (8)	Breathing (1) Present Moment (8)
LUNCH	LUNCH	LUNCH	LUNCH
Breathing (1) Standing Breathing (4)		Breathing (1)	
DINNER	DINNER	DINNER	DINNER
Decision (5) Clearing (2)	Decision (5) Clearing (2)	Pebble (6) Decision (5) Clearing (2)	Decision (5) Clearing (2)

Day 14 SUNDAY	Day 15 MONDAY	Day 16 TUESDAY
Decision (5) Standing Breathing (4)	Decision (5) Mirror (7)	Decision (5)
BREAKFAST	**BREAKFAST**	**BREAKFAST**
Breathing (1) Present Moment (8) Standing Breathing (4)	Breathing (1) Present Moment (8)	Breathing (1) Present Moment (8)
LUNCH	**LUNCH**	**LUNCH**
Standing Breathing (4)	Breathing (1)	Breathing (1)
DINNER	**DINNER**	**DINNER**
Decision (5) Clearing (2)	Decision (5) Clearing (2)	Decision (5) Clearing (2)

Key to numbers:
(1) Breathing practice
(2) Clearing exercise
(3) Rejuvenation exercise (whenever needed)
(4) Breathing practice (standing)
(5) Decision exercise
(6) Pebble in the water exercise
(7) Mirror exercise
(8) Present Moment exercise

Day 17 WEDNESDAY	Day 18 THURSDAY	Day 19 FRIDAY	Day 20 SATURDAY
Decision (5) Standing Breathing (4)	Decision (5)	Decision (5)	Decision (5)
BREAKFAST	BREAKFAST	BREAKFAST	BREAKFAST
Breathing (1) Present Moment (8) Standing Breathing (4)	Breathing (1) Present Moment (8)	Breathing (1) Present Moment (8)	Breathing (1) Present Moment (8)
LUNCH	LUNCH	LUNCH	LUNCH
Breathing (1) Standing Breathing (4)		Breathing (1)	
DINNER	DINNER	DINNER	DINNER
Decision (5) Clearing (2)	Decision (5) Clearing (2)	Pebble (6) Decision (5) Clearing (2)	Decision (5) Clearing (2)

Day 21 SUNDAY	Day 22 MONDAY	Day 23 TUESDAY
Decision (5) Standing Breathing (4)	Decision (5) Mirror (7)	Decision (5)
BREAKFAST	BREAKFAST	BREAKFAST
Breathing (1) Present Moment (8) Standing Breathing (4)	Breathing (1) Present Moment (8)	Breathing (1) Present Moment (8)
LUNCH	LUNCH	LUNCH
Standing Breathing (4)	Breathing (1)	Breathing (1)
DINNER	DINNER	DINNER
Decision (5) Clearing (2)	Pebble (6) Decision (5) Clearing (2)	Decision (5) Clearing (2)

Key to numbers:
(1) Breathing practice
(2) Clearing exercise
(3) Rejuvenation exercise (whenever needed)
(4) Breathing practice (standing)

(5) Decision exercise
(6) Pebble in the water exercise
(7) Mirror exercise
(8) Present Moment exercise

Day 24

WEDNESDAY	THURSDAY	FRIDAY
Decision (5) Standing Breathing (4) Mirror (7)		
BREAKFAST	BREAKFAST	BREAKFAST
Breathing (1) Present Moment (8) Standing Breathing (4)	Breathing (1)	Breathing (1)
LUNCH	LUNCH	LUNCH
Breathing (1) Standing Breathing (4)		Breathing (1)
DINNER	DINNER	DINNER
Pebble (6) Decision (5) Clearing (2)		

Epilogue

The intention of this book has been to open up possibilities for those who wish to be able to better serve their fellow creatures and the planet itself. Although some of the ideas may have sounded far-fetched, their practical application is essentially simple. The practices suggested for the twenty-four day cycle can be undertaken by virtually anyone. If the purpose of the task is continually remembered, and the intention firmly set at the beginning, resistance to the disciplines involved will soon melt away as the programme unfolds and greater confidence will be felt.

Indeed, now is a time of great change and we need all the help we can get. I pray that this book will have opened up uncharted shores for many of you, and confirmed the feelings and intuitions of others.

May all be well!

Santa Cruz, California
April 1 1985

The Invisible Way

A Time to Love – A Time to Die

Reshad Feild

A beautiful and moving story about Reshad Feild's quest for inner understanding and a sequel to his first book *The Last Barrier*. It begins with recollections of experiences in Mexico, Turkey and Konya. Returning to his teacher an all-surmounting wish is revealed to him: 'I need to know that I am loved.' For surely in finding that profundity of love, would he not then begin to know the source of love itself?

This revelation provides the key to the doors which open to him on his return to London, bringing new contacts which mysteriously link with past acquaintances and situations. Among these is Nur – the young woman with whom he shares a bond of a quality which is new to him. With her he is to share experiences which deepen his understanding of life, death and love. He also discovers a new dimension to the role of woman.

'Best of all, it filled me with great joy and singing. And gratitude.'
TINA MORRIS *Resurgence*

187 pages 216 x 138mm ISBN 0 906540 04 6 £5.50 *net*

Steps to Freedom

Discourses on the Alchemy of the Heart

Reshad Feild

These are discourses on the essential knowledge of the heart, about being in such a state of love that we come to understand the perfection of life in each moment. Reshad's first two books, *The Last Barrier* and *The Invisible Way,* are already classics of contemporary spiritual literature. This third book of the trilogy explicitly develops the transformative ideas that made the first two books so powerful and popular. Developing will, asking the question, making love, serving the Guest, breath, the path of return, brotherhood.

160 pages 210 x 134mm ISBN 0 939660 04 0 *paperback* £6.95

The Last Barrier

Reshad Feild

Here is a rare journal of one man's struggle towards true freedom.
An exciting story, it carries the stamp of undeniable authenticity.
Reshad Feild chose the Sufi way of enlightenment, but *The Last
Barrier* in essence is the universal search for self-discovery.

"Order and perfection seem to be the keynotes of Mr. Feild's
message. His eloquent and colourful orchestration ... shows his
creative powers to be of a very high level."
The Times Literary Supplement

"The author places himself firmly in the tradition of many of
mankind's greatest teachers. Those who are entering upon the life
of the Spirit will surely gain from this book."
Radionic Quarterly

"The first of a trilogy of a genuine Spiritual Quest."
Evening Press Dublin

183 *pages 7 line drawings*
216 x 138*mm* ISBN 0 906540 52 6 *paperback* £5.50